Elderly Widows

Elderly Widows

Socio-economic and Demographic Study in Jharkhand

Sangeeta Gupta

RAWAT PUBLICATIONS

Jaipur • New Delhi • Bangalore • Guwahati • Kolkata

ISBN 978-81-316-0870-8

The publication of this book was financially supported by the ICSSR. The responsibility for the facts stated, opinions expressed, or conclusions reached, is entirely that of the author and that the ICSSR accepts no responsibility for them.

ICSSR Consultant: Professor P.M. Kulkarni, Centre for Study of Regional Development (CSRD), Jawaharlal Nehru University, New Delhi.

Published by
Prem Rawat for **Rawat Publications**
Satyam Apts., Sector 3, Jawahar Nagar, Jaipur 302 004 (India)
Phone: 0141 265 1748 / 7006 Fax: 0141 265 1748
E-mail: info@rawatbooks.com
Website: www.rawatbooks.com

New Delhi Office
4858/24, Ansari Road, Daryaganj, New Delhi 110 002
Phone: 011-23263290

Also at *Bangalore, Guwahati* and *Kolkata*

Printed at Nice Printing Press, New Delhi

Contents

List of Tables, Maps and Figures

Tables

Maps

Figures

Acknowledgements

It gives me immense pleasure to acknowledge the help, support, encouragement, assistance and guidance of all those who have made it possible for me to complete this research work.

At the outset, I would like to express the most sincere thanks and profound sense of gratitude and indebtedness to my research guide Dr T.V. Sekher, Professor, Department of Population Policies and Programmes, International Institute for Population Sciences (IIPS), for his valuable suggestions, encouragement, patience, cooperation and guidance. His involvement with my work right from the beginning has helped me to complete the work successfully. He not only facilitated my research and encouraged all my endeavours, but also provided me constant moral support. I am greatly indebted to him for the support throughout my Ph.D. work.

I also express my sincere thanks to my advisory committee members, Dr B. Paswan, Professor, Department of Population Policies and Programmes, IIPS; and Dr Chander Shekhar, Professor, Department of Mathematical Demography and Statistics, IIPS – for their suggestions and encouragement that helped me a lot at different stages of this research work.

I owe my gratitude to Prof. F. Ram, Director and Senior Professor, IIPS, for providing me the opportunity to undertake this work and also his constant encouragement and support during my Ph.D. work.

I wish to thank all faculty members of IIPS for their encouragement and support throughout the study. I am obliged to Dr

S.K. Mohanty, Professor, Department of Fertility Studies, and Dr Aparajita Chattopadhyay, Assistant Professor, Department of Development Studies, IIPS, for fruitful suggestions during my research proposal presentation. I am deeply grateful to Dr T.K. Roy, Retired Professor, IIPS, for providing me valuable suggestions during the development of questionnaire for data collection.

I am thankful to Dr Sayeed Unisa, Professor, Department of Mathematical Demography and Statistics, for her affection, support, motivation and encouragement throughout my work. I owe my gratitude to Prof. Sulabha Parasuraman, Retired Professor, IIPS; Dr R.B. Bhagat, Professor, Department of Migration Studies; Dr P. Arokiasamy, Professor, Department of Development Studies; Dr S.K. Singh, Professor, Department of Mathematical Demography and Statistics; Dr Usha Ram, Professor, Department of Public Health and Mortality Studies; Dr Manoj Alagarajan, Assistant Professor, Department of Development Studies; and Dr Abhishek Singh, Associate Professor, Department of Public Health and Mortality Studies, for their incessant support and words of encouragement during my research work.

I am also thankful to the International Institute on Ageing (United Nations), Malta, for selecting me to be a part of their training programme on 'Social Gerontology', which provided me an opportunity to familiarize with this theme, and the International Summer School, University of Oslo, Norway, for giving me the chance to understand the recent global developments and emerging issues in the developing countries. I also had the opportunity to present the findings of this study in various national and international conferences, including the conference of the Asian Population Association (APA) in 2010.

I acknowledge the help and cooperation extended by Mr M. Sekar, Assistant Registrar (Academic), IIPS, throughout my Ph.D. work. I also acknowledge the support and cooperation I have received from the staff members of Academic Section – Mr Somnath Chougle, Mr Ankush, Mrs Dhanlaxmi, Mrs P. Swant and Mr Tilak throughout my study period.

The contribution and assistance received at various stages of this work from Mr D.D. Mestry, Library and Information Officer

(IIPS), Mr Praveen Kumar, Assistant Library and Information Officer. Mr Vidhate, Mr Vasu, Mr Santosh, Mr Aashish, Mr Rakesh, Mr Sudhir and all others deserve special mention. I am very thankful to Prof. M. Guruswamy, and Prof. S. Unisa, Computer Centre in-charge, and all the staff members of Computer Centre, for providing necessary digital assistance and support during my research work.

I am indebted to Prof. B. Paswan and Prof. T.V. Sekher (Hostel Wardens) for providing me hostel accommodation during my Ph.D. tenure.

The Doctoral Fellowship from the Government of India has been invaluable to successfully complete my research work.

I cannot forget the immense help and active support received from Mr Seshnath Roy (District Co-ordinator, UNICEF) for helping me in identification of surveyed villages. I express my deep gratitude to Mr Amar Kumar (Block Development Officer, Baharagora), Ms Praveena Soren (Block Programme Officer, Baharagora), Mr Sudeep Das (Block Co-ordinator, UNICEF), Mr Om Prakash Kumar (Block Development Officer, Ghatshila) for providing me important information and also supporting me whenever I needed help during the field work. I express my sincere thanks to Mr Ravi Nath Das (Mukhiya of Baharagora village) and Mrs Reena, Mrs Bimala, Mrs Shanti, Mrs Krisana, Mrs Pushpa, Mrs Veronika, Ms Kajal, Ms Vandana, Ms Deepti, and Mr Tapan Rawat, for providing me necessary local support during the data collection.

I cannot afford to forget the immense support, encouragement and help received from Ms Priti Devi Verma during my data collection. She made my stay convenient and without her co-operation and active support, it would have been difficult to complete the field work.

I express my sincere thanks to my seniors, specially Mrs Soumya Praharaj, for their suggestions and support during the drafting questionnaire and during various stages of my research work. I would also like to thank my friends, for their co-operation during my work.

I am grateful to my Dada ji, my father, my sisters – Kavita, Sarita and Preeti, my brother, my sister-in-law, my brother-in-law, Praveen Srivastava, and other family members, who provided constant support, love and affection, even though I was far away from my home, whenever I needed it the most. They took a lot of pain in helping me cross all hurdles while carrying out this research work. I owe my sincere thanks to Mithlesh bhaiya for his help, support and encouragement during my research work. There are no words to express my admiration for my husband Anupam Gupta and his family members. Their immense support, love and motivation have always been a source of encouragement to complete this work successfully.

I have no words to express the feelings of gratitude and obligation towards my beloved mother for the inspiration which gave me strength to complete this work successfully, even though she is not with us to see the Ph.D. thesis. I dedicate this work to her sacred memory.

I am thankful to Indian Council of Social Science Research (ICSSR) for awarding the publication grant which facilitated in the publication of this book. My thanks are also due to Rawat Publications, Jaipur, for publishing this book.

Last, but not the least, my very special thanks to all my elderly respondents for their co-operation during field work without which I could not have completed this Ph.D. work. It was really a learning experience for me by interacting closely with many senior citizens. I am sorry, if I have missed out anyone but all of you mean a lot to me.

Sangeeta Kumari Gupta

1

Introduction and Review of Literature

The ageing of a population is an outcome of an increase in the proportion of the aged *vis-a-vis* a decrease in the proportion of the young. Improved life expectancy has given rise to an increase in the number of persons aged 60 years and above. In 1950, the proportion of elder persons in the world was around 8 per cent and it has increased to 10 per cent in 2000 and projected to reach 21 per cent by 2050. It is estimated that the elderly population will reach almost 1.2 billion by 2025 and 2 billion by 2050 (United Nations, 2002). According to United Nations (2006), one out of every 10 persons in the world now is an elderly (60 years and above).

Population ageing is a world-wide phenomenon. India is no exception to this global phenomenon of ageing even with the modest decline in fertility and mortality levels. The Indian aged population is currently the second largest in the world. The absolute number of the 60+ population in India will increase from 77 million in 2001 to 137 million by 2021 (United Nations, 2002). Owing to the longer life expectancy of females, it is expected that in the coming years the majority of the older persons will be women. The Census of India indicates that the 60+ category favoured the males, but in the 70+ age group, the ratio of females is higher than males, which is explained by the higher life expectancy at age 60+ for females in comparison to males. One of the main social effects of extension of life is the extended period of widowhood for many Indian women.

Table 1.1

Life Expectancy at Birth, at Ages 60 and 70 years for Males and Females, India

Year	Males			Females		
	e0	e60	e70	e0	e60	e70
1970–75	50.5	13.4	8.6	49.0	14.3	9.2
1976–80	52.5	14.1	9.6	52.1	15.9	10.9
1981–85	55.5	14.6	9.7	55.7	16.4	11.0
1986–90	57.7	14.7	9.4	58.1	16.1	10.1
1991–95	59.7	15.3	10.0	60.9	17.1	11.0
1995–99	60.8	15.7	10.3	62.5	17.7	11.6
2001–05	62.3	16.4	10.9	63.9	18.7	12.3
2002–06	62.6	16.7	10.9	64.2	18.9	12.4

Source: SRS Based Abridged Life Tables, Registrar General of India (various years)

According to 2001 Census, there are 34 million widows in India constituting 6 per cent of the total female population and 52 per cent of the women over the age of 60 years. According to NSSO (60th Round), there were 62 widows and 22 widowers per 100 old persons (60 and above years) in rural areas. The respective figures were 38 and 10 for urban areas. In other words, more than 50 per cent of elder women in India live without a spouse as compared to only 20 per cent of elder men. There are three reasons for this gender disparity in widowhood in India – longer life span of women than that of men, the general tendency for men to marry women younger than themselves, and the higher rate of remarriage among widowed men compared to that among widowed women.

In spite of the socio-economic changes in Indian society over the decades, the position of women has not improved much. Even in family, they are mostly dependents throughout their life. Widowhood is the drastic change in the status of women brought out by the death of the spouse and this necessitates the establishment of new support within the family, within the kin-group and within the community. Widowhood is characterized as one of the most distressing of all life events (Holmes and Rahe, 1967). Mostly, widowhood implies a shift in position from that of a wife with economic, social and emotional security to that of socially and financially insecure women. For many women, '*widowhood is more than the loss of a husband – it may mean the loss of a separate identity*' (UNFPA, 1998: 42).

Status of Women and Widows in India: Historical Perspectives

Traditionally, women had a unique position in the Indian culture. During the *Pre-Vedic* times, women were adored as a deity and an incarnation of *Shakti* (energy). She was treated with respect and occupied an important place in almost all social and religious functions.

During the *Vedic* period, women had equal rights with men, and in all respects were their equal partners and friends. During this period, women could remarry and start a new life. '*Niyoga*' was a social custom allowing a widow or even a woman with her living husband, to have children through men other than her husband. '*Satidaha*' (widow dying along with her husband) was not in vogue during the *Vedic* age. Moreover, widows had full rights to perform all religious activities and enjoyed equal rights as the widowers. Women in *Vedic* period had equal rights as men to own property.

The Epic Age too (500 BC+), like the Vedic age, was known for its beneficial treatment of women. But, during this period, the status of women was not as good as during the *Vedic* age. Women could choose their partners freely through '*swayamvara-vratha*' (freedom of choice) and marriage was not compulsory. Women's contribution to fields of education and culture were of a high order. But, the deteriorating process had started after *Vedic* age and its mark was first found in the sphere of women's rights and privileges.

During the *Smriti* Age (AD 500+), there was a big change. Women who rose to the heights of knowledge and realization, who vied with men in all spheres of life and even surpassed them in many spheres, who enjoyed full freedom and equal rights with men in self-dependence, self-determination, and who were self-confident and self-relying, were gradually confined within the four walls of the household (Jamuna, 2008). They became depressed, with many of their rights substantially curtailed in such things as justice in education, equality in the domestic, social, legal, economic and political spheres. Men considered women in marriage only for the purpose of procreation, which resulted in the emergence of social customs for women, e.g. girl-gifting (in marriage), *'satidahana'* or widow-burning, *'vidhava-pirana'* or widow-baiting (Altekar, 1973).

It was stated in *Manusmriti* that the father protects a women during her childhood; husband during her youth and the sons during her old age. Thus, a woman does not deserve freedom but protection and dependency. She just has to play certain roles and no opportunity is given to her to take decisions and to act on her own. This clearly shows how the status of women had deteriorated from the *Vedic* to the *Smriti* ages (Indira, 1955). In the late 19th and early 20th centuries, efforts for the betterment of women were undertaken. Since Independence, many steps to raise their overall status have been introduced in India.

Despite the increasing education and improved technology, the familial position of the women does not seem to have undergone any radical change. The Indian culture has strongly emphasized feminine fertility. It has been stressed that a women is not to outlive the husband and that she should be fortunate to die before the death of her husband. As a result, there is a strong stigma attached both to widowhood and sterility among the women (Karve, 1968). These historical facts have invariably contributed to the difficulties the women of today is likely to encounter during the post-fertility period and particularly if she were to lose her husband. Both tradition and the scriptures were not in favour of widow remarriage. They placed severe restrictions on the social and familial roles of widows (Jamuna, 2008). Until recently, women did not have equal property rights with men. Despite increasing education and continuing attempts for social reforms, the position of elderly women or elderly widows are not very encouraging. This is more so in the rural areas. To some extent, younger generation of women is having the benefit of education and modernization. However, many of the elderly widows have faced the storms of family life and strains of living (Prakash, 1996).

In India, the social structure is constituted of classes defined in relation to their role in social production in the background of caste. Castes accentuate class exploitation through mythical and religious legitimization. Women being subject to such exploitation are deprived of and oppressed on the basis of gender discrimination and widowhood (Halạkatti, 1988).

> A widow is supposed to be disfigured; her ornaments are removed, her heads shaved, and she has to dress white sari. After that she is expected to give up eating 'hot' foods, to avoid auspicious occasions because she is considered inauspicious and to remain celibate, devout and loyal to her husband. (Chen, 1998: 26)

Hindu society over the centuries encouraged the practices of female infanticide, child marriage, *sati* and *purdah* system and also discouraged female education. Among the upper caste women, *sati* became a mark of prestige. The natural affection towards the husband became a forceful and obligatory action. Social evils like *sati*, problems of widowhood, female infanticide, *purdah* system, dowry, child marriage, polyandry, *devadasi* system, etc. had infected the society badly. *Sati* was prevalent among the high castes. Those women who saved themselves from *sati* somehow had to live a life, which was more miserable than self-immolation. Self-immolation was momental suffering, but widowhood was a life-long suffering (Thara Bhai, 2004).

The presence of social evils was a major hindrance to the society's development. Many progressive measures were introduced by the British government. This period of British rule was referred to as 'Social Reform Era'. Raja Ram Mohan Roy saw his sister-in-law's self-immolation on the funeral of his brother. At that time he made up his mind to get this inhuman practice of *sati* abolished. He got *sati* completely abolished with the help of Lord Bentinck in 1829 by passing of the 'Decree for the Abolition of Sati'. In 1856, the traditional Hindu ban on widow remarriage was also overturned by law with passing of the Widow Remarriage Act by the efforts made by social reformers like Ishwar Chandra Vidyasagar and Keshab Chandra Sen. They worked for the upliftment of women and the first widow remarriage was performed under their inspiration in 1864.

Widow Remarriage in India: An Overview

The attitude towards remarriage of widows has varied from time to time. In the age of Rig Veda and later Samhitas, Brahmanas and Upanishads, remarriage of widows are permitted. Later, widow remarriage was discouraged by upper castes. There may be two possible reasons to discourage the widow remarriage – possibility of conflicting claims of children from two marriages and the other more important reason was a belief that marriage may be sustained into next cycle of life (Reddy, 1988).

However, remarriage among the widows of lower castes does take place. Widow remarriage is still permissible among all the tribal communities (Sarkar and Banerjee, 1998). In more traditional societies, the system of levirate made it possible for a widow to marry one of the brothers of the dead husband, especially in north India. Using the 1971 Census data, Bhat and Kanbargi (1984) have estimated that about 34 per cent of widows and 63 per cent of widowers were remarried. They have also estimated the absolute number of remarried widows as 12 million and remarried widowers as 14 million in 1971.

Census Report of 1911 (Mysore) states that the marriage of widows is prohibited only among Brahmins and in a very few other castes. Nair (1978), in his study, illustrated that widow remarriage is universal among the tribal people of India and the proper groom is her younger brother-in-law. A person who wishes to marry a widow has to return the bride-price to the deceased husband's family, in case the widow marries to an outsider. A similar conclusion is drawn by Bose (1966) who found that widow remarriage is not only prevalent in rural areas but it is even encouraged, especially among lower castes. However, it was prohibited among Rajput, Brahmin, Purohit and Mahajan castes of north India.

Baron and Ehrenfels (1941) found that in Kerala, a negative marriage is in practice. Under this practice a widow is allowed to marry other than the brother-in-law. In Karnataka, though the widow remarriage is in practice among certain lower castes, there are certain restrictions on the choice of the groom. The Bedas, Okkaliggas, Holeyas, Madigas, Vaddas, Vayindas, Mandas, Dasari, Bilimagga, Uppars and many castes do not permit the widow marriage with the brother-in-law. The Bedas, Madigas, Bilimagga, Sanyasi, and Uppars allow the widow to marry within the close circle of husband's *Kula* (Patil, 2000).

Though the widow remarriage is allowed, the widows receive less encouragement than widowers to remarry. The majority of women are widowed at an advanced age, and thus it is difficult for them to change the status through remarriage (Duval, 1971). Hence proportionately more widowers than widows remarry. Though remarriage is the most satisfactory adjustment to widowhood, this practice among widows depends upon several conditions like:

(1) *Duration of widowhood:* Recently widowed have greater chances than those bereaved much earlier.
(2) *Number of children:* There is a co-relation between the chances of remarriage and the number of children. More number of children, lesser the chances of remarriage.
(3) *Widow's pension:* The widow who receives the pension that terminates upon remarriage may be unwilling to forfeit this benefit (Truxual and Merrill, 1953).

The negative attitude towards remarriage of widows is so strong that even today people believe that this practice does not have either social or religious sanction. Srinivas (1982) stated that the reason for the negative attitude towards widows' remarriage is due to Sanskritic civilization, the non-Brahmin wish to rise in the social scale by imitating Brahmin customs and ceremonies.

Problems of Widows and Widowhood

The caring for the elderly in the past was not considered a serious issue in India as they were provided with social protection, mostly in the joint family living arrangements. Studies revealed that women suffer from different kinds of eventualities in their old age (Dandekar, 1986; Rajan et al., 1999). The changes in demographic parameters influence the health, economic activity and social conditions of the people. As the age structure of developing countries changes, demands on resources by different segments of population also expected to grow. There are many priorities that may push the interests of the elderly to the background. Ageing itself has major socio-economic implications, but when ageing is combined with being widowed, another important dimension is added.

In India's traditional rural set-up, widowhood is both a crisis and a problem. When it occurs, its suddenness and intensity make it a crisis and as the individual finds ways of coping, it becomes a problem. Widowhood brings about both subjective and objective consequences. The subjective consequences can be almost the same for widows and widowers, but objective consequences differ due to the distinctively different roles of men and women (Radha Devi, 1987). The major role of the man is that of a provider and of woman as a home-maker. When death strikes the spouse, a man loses a home-maker, but a woman loses a provider. Hence, widow faces a much more serious situation than the widower.

Many times, a widow faces difficulty in adjusting to her new status because the social norms and taboos place her in most disadvantaged position and restrict her social interactions. A widow has to perform many rituals. She has to follow lot many restrictions leading to social isolation and social inferiority, resulting in a feeling of dejection and depression. Widows in all communities suffer from limited freedom to participate in religious and social functions. They carry the stigma of inauspicious and hence have to keep away from functions. For instance, they are not allowed to touch objects used during marriage or religious ceremonies. In fact, a widow is not even entitled to perform the ritual to welcome her own daughter-in-law (Sarkar and Banerjee, 1998).

Kelphart (1981) argues that widowhood is a problem of many dimensions; numerical, financial and emotional. Widowhood also brings about a variety of social problems related to adult and child dependency, poverty, unemployment, illness, family disorganization, and women's insecure status. Widows face negative, long-term and severe problems and these seem to be derived from social, economic, cultural and emotional deprivations than from the widowhood itself. One of the immediate problems following widowhood is economic dispossession. Widowed women in traditional societies often face a sudden change in status and limited life choices. Widowed women's life could be highly disrupted if she does not have economic means of support (Parvathy, 2004). With the advancing of age and deterioration in health, it is generally accepted that one's ability to support oneself economically is reduced and consequently one becomes dependent on others (Gulati, 1998).

There are several demographic, economic, social and psychological consequences of widowhood. Demographic consequences of widowhood will be mainly on the rate of population growth, fertility behaviour, and number of eligible women available for marriage in different age groups. Social consequences are many. In traditional societies like ours, women derive her social status from her husband. The death of her husband not only disrupts her social environment but also her kinship relationship. She feels out of place in her in-laws' as well as in parents' house and in addition to this, she is not accustomed from the beginning to lead an independent life.

Psychological consequences are equally unfavourable to the widowed. Loneliness and depression may lead to mental disorder. Aged widows suffer higher incidences of mental disorder because of the greater isolation and feeling of insecurity. They have to adjust to the settings in changed social environment. Alone they have to cope up with decline in functional capacity and well-being.

Problems of Elderly Widows

The impact of widowhood is not equally felt by all age groups. However, like cultural variants, age also has an important role. It is observed that a younger widow learns faster to adjust to a life without a spouse (Green, 1977). She establishes new friendship more easily and discovers novel ways to integrate herself in the wider community, than her elderly counterpart for whom widowhood is a critical situation which entails both social and personal disorganization. Additionally, socio-economic factors like poverty, lack of economic independence, and inheritance system depriving women from property rights worsen the position of Indian widows which further leads them to a feeling of great insecurity and stress (Mehta et al., 2006). The widowed condition places women in a more disadvantaged position in their old age and they live as dependents for a long time. Elder widows are doubly affected due to the combined effects of old age and widowhood.

Elder widows, because of their high level of economic dependency, are vulnerable to abuse from family and also from society. Widowhood becomes intolerable to women who lack both economic and social support. Most of the older women in India have no old age pension or any form of social security, except the support from children or relatives (Shankardass, 2003).

The elderly married males enjoy better health than the elderly females (Bose and Gangrade, 1988). This is largely due to the traditional role that women play as the prime care-givers, coupled with the lower status they enjoy, which leaves them with limited access to financial resources. Consequently, the health of the elderly women gets ignored, which is further aggravated by the stigma of widowhood. Due to various socio-cultural and economic reasons, widows are in a vulnerable position.

Law and Property Rights of Widows in India

There is no uniform law in India governing the rights of widows to inherit property-movable or immovable. Property rights and inheritance are governed by the personal laws of each religious community. Among the Hindus, there are two kinds of property – ancestral/joint family property and self-acquired property. Traditionally, there were two schools of law governing ancestral property: the *Dayabhaga* and the *Mitakshara*. According to the *Mitakshara* law, a male member of the joint family had a right by birth in the ancestral property. Women did not have any right by birth in the ancestral property. They were only entitled to expenses incurred for their food, shelter, clothing, education and marriage out of such property.

The Hindu Succession Act, 1956, brought about a number of changes. A Hindu male could now will away his interest in the ancestral property. If a man died intestate, his share would be divided amongst his heirs. His heirs would be his sons, daughters, widows, mother, children of a predeceased son or a predeceased daughter, and widowed daughter-in-law. Under the

Hindu Succession Act, women became absolute owners of the property they inherited. Under the Mohammedan law of inheritance, a male could only will away one-third of his property. A widow is entitled to one-eighth of her husband's property if there were children and one-fourth if there were no children. If a man had two or more widows, together they would inherit one-eighth or one-fourth share, depending on whether he had children or not.

Although laws exist in the Hindu and other religious communities, does the actual practice reflect these or not? To investigate the societal perceptions about the property rights for the widows, a study (Misra and Thukral, 1998) in the two villages in Bihar found that all widows, irrespective of caste or economic background, felt that they are the rightful heir to their husband's share of the property but they did not have the real control over it. Whether they could actually exercise their rights depends on a number of factors, including the age of the widow, whether she had children, the sex and age of the children, the status of her parental family, the attitude of her in-laws, whether the land had been partitioned before the husband's death, whether the widow remarried, and where she lived. Further, it was also mentioned by one of the widows in the study that *'if we want to sell the property, the unwritten rule is that we have to first ask our brother-in-law to buy it'* (p. 245). Thus, it is fairly clear that while in practice, both the society and the women themselves saw the widows as having a right to a share in the husband's property, but in practice these rights were limited and restricted.

Kodoth and Rajan (2008) found that widowed persons, irrespective of their sex, have lower incidence of ownership of property and assets and also lower participation in the management of property. In rural India, more than 80 per cent of aged men and 48 per cent of aged women own property, whereas only 44 per cent of aged widows and 74 per cent of aged widowers do so.

Review of Literature

Marital status of the elderly assumes special significance in the context of care in old age as it is known that those who are married fare better in all economic and social aspects than those who remain single. Though there are many studies on elderly in

India, very few attempted to focus on elderly widows. In every age group, women experience more widowhood than men and in the middle-age group, nearly three times more than men.

A survey on elderly in Kerala (Rajan et al., 1999) observed that a higher proportion of older women live more than 10 years as widows. Widowhood influences the economic status of older women because they lack the opportunity to benefit from their spouse's earnings. Dreze and Srinivasan (1997), based on the National Sample Survey data on consumer expenditure, examined the relationship between widowhood and poverty in rural India and found that widows are no more likely to live in poverty than non-widows, but because widows tend to live in households with fewer members, even small adjustments for economies of scale result in widows being significantly worse off than average.

Kitchlu's (1993) study among the widows from urban and rural areas of Delhi found that 78 per cent of the widows started working after the death of their husbands due to sheer economic necessity. Among rural widows, 30 per cent faced problem in getting jobs in comparison to 14 per cent of urban widows who had better educational attainment. Further, it was also found that the rural widows mostly depend on their own earnings or that of their children or if they work, generally work on the farm of the joint family or take up some casual work. A good number of urban widows were interested in doing some remunerative work to support their families.

In India, family is the most important traditional social institution, where everybody gets shelter and care whether it is a child, youth, disabled, ill, elderly, or widow. The family serves as a fundamental structure for living together intimately and sharing economic, social and emotional responsibilities. Family as an intimate group provides protection to the sick, economically inactive and the aged. Security and emotional satisfaction to the individual can be provided through a network of inter-personal relations, implicit reciprocal duties and obligations between the family members. But the structural changes that have been taking place in the society and the gradual disintegration of the joint family system, is resulting in the rejection and neglect of the aged.

A study in Delhi (Soodan, 1975) revealed that 80 per cent of the elderly widows were living with their sons. About one-half of the widows who do not have sons were staying with their married daughters, whereas about 10 per cent reported to be living alone. Audinarayana et al. (1997), in a study in rural Tamil Nadu, observed that elderly women/widowed tend to live substantially in large numbers as a single member family than that of men. The possible reasons – not getting support from son(s), son(s) living in nearby towns for work, reluctant to live with married daughter, and adjustment problems or strained relations with daughter(s)-in-law.

Aruna and Reddy (2001) in their study on sibling relationships in widowhood found that young widows with unmarried female children receive significantly greater support from brothers. Widows who have small land holdings receive very little support in comparison to those with large land holdings.

Martin and Preston (1994) argued that the living arrangements among the elderly are mainly influenced by the size and composition of their kin networks. The size of the household is a good indicator of the familial well-being. Living arrangements are associated with the level of care and assistance received by the elderly. If more and more people are living together, the elderly are likely to get better attention, including care during sickness (Prasad, 2007). Comparing the gender differentials in family structure and related aspects, Audinarayana et al. (1997) found that the family support and care for elderly women are relatively less than elderly men. In rural Maharashtra, majority of the elderly women stated that children do not take care of their aged parents. The oldest-old elderly (80+ years) from low economic status are more likely to have negative perceptions towards younger generation (Bansod, 2007).

While comparing the living arrangements among the married women and widowed Audinarayana and Kavitha (1997) found that living arrangements of the elderly women are highly associated with number of living rooms in the house and per capita family income per adult. In case of widowed women, number of surviving sons exhibited a positive association with the living arrangements of the elderly. Based on NFHS data,

Rajan and Kumar (2003) found that 80 per cent of the elderly lives with their adult children. This is even more in the case of elderly widows. Further, males were much more likely to have the status of head of the intergenerational households than elderly women, and if the women are heading the household, then it is often because they are destitute widows or living alone. Living alone implies coping with illness harder than living with other individuals.

The change in the living arrangements may be related to economic factors for the widows. Among the elderly living with their adult children, majority were found to be either totally or partially dependent upon their children for economic need. Even if a widow lives as a dependent in a household headed by others, she is likely to be subjected to neglect, unless she is seen to contribute something important to the household. For example contribution through domestic services, land or other property, wage earnings or a pension, which reflect inherent weaknesses in traditional family and community-based forms of social security (Chen, 1998).

Singh's (1986) study on 'Problems of Widowhood' found that about 85 per cent of widows faced variety of financial problems. A study on Kashivasi widows observed that more than half of the widows received no economic support from their parents or husband's family (Saraswati, 1988). About 60 per cent of widows living in the joint families left their homes under compelling and painful circumstances. A majority of the relatives do not visit the widows. These painful experiences within the family seem to be a contributing factor for most widows for not maintaining any contact with family members.

Nandlal et al. (1987) argued that the elderly who handed over their property to their children lost on their role as decision-makers. They observed that elderly females suffer the loss of status more than the elderly males. Sureender et al. (1996) illustrate the status of widows in rural Tamil Nadu, especially their involvement in social functions and their role in decision-making at the family level. They observed that in general, rural widows are not invited to any of the social functions and the treatment given to them is intolerable. Another study

(Thara Bhai, 2004) found that 75 per cent of widows felt change in their life after the death of their husbands. Widows feel that their status depends upon the attitude towards them by the members of the immediate society. It was also found that the power of the women in the family changed after the death of their husbands and the decision-making control was taken over by other male members of the family. Even the economically independent widow has no authority in the house as other members took the decisions on her behalf.

Female elderly, especially widows, lack access to and control over productive resources such as land may be because of patrilineal and patrilocal societal arrangements which make them more vulnerable. Bhat (1992) argued that the demographic trends in India call for a rapid expansion of public support systems for the elderly. In Bangladesh, the social role of elderly women changes from the head of the domestic realm to that of the quiet and unassuming 'old widows', indicating the loss of authority and status for most widows (Ellickson, 1988).

Martin (1989) has observed that significant changes in the familial relations of elderly may take place with an increasing age, deteriorating health, the diminishing job opportunities, especially when an economic loss is involved. The family members and the society may feel the burden of taking care of the elderly when the elderly are unable to participate in economic activities, including the increasing cost for health care. The health of the elderly women gets ignored and further aggravated by the stigma of widowhood. Mini (2009) while analysing the socio-economic and demographic diversity in the health status of the elderly in Kerala found that among the female elderly, marital status, place of residence, religion and work status are having significant relationship with their health status. Study by Sheoran et al., in Hayrana (2004) observed that majority of aged widows (63%) had impaired health status. Sometimes to avoid financial burden on the family, elders usually ignore regular health treatment. One-third of the aged widows relied on others for financial support at the time of illness. Few spent their own savings, some ignored medical treatment and one per cent took support from daughters.

Indian widow tends to be a highly marginalized person. She typically receives very little support from persons other than her own children and even when she lives with her adult sons she remains highly vulnerable to neglect (Sivagami and Thamilrasan, 2004). About one-third of the elderly were at risk of economic and social problems due to widowhood, highlighting the extent of vulnerability (Panda, 1994; Kumari and Sekher, 2010).

A study in Andhra Pradesh by Lalitha and Jamuna (2004), on the social problems of adjustment among widows and widowers, indicated that widows report more number of problems of adjustment than widowers. The problems of adjustments shows that widows reported high intensity of problems in the areas of health and economic aspects and widowers had high intensity of problems in the areas of self and emotions. Widows perceived stress from family responsibilities and experienced psychological problems heavily but none of them opted for remarriage (Kumari, 2004). Further it was found that the feeling of helplessness, difficulty in making decisions, and stress due to increased responsibilities are more among widows.

The findings of Aggarwal and Chadha (1990) indicated that married elderly found to be low on hopelessness and high on life satisfaction as compared to widow/widower. Balachandran et al. (2007) studied the life satisfaction and alienation among the elderly males and females and found that the elderly women show more alienation than elderly men. A study by Pandya and Shah (2006) analysed the problems reported by the widows and observed that more than one-fourth of the widows had psychological problems which includes isolation, feeling of loneliness, helplessness, alienation, lack of support, and lack of encouragement. Sijuwade's (2008) study found that religion is an important instrument for the individual to console with emotionally distressful life situations.

Aruna and Reddy (2001) studied the social relations of widows in their day-to-day life and examined which relationships provide what kind of support in the dimensions of emotional and financial services. Study found that immediate kin are the most available source in all spheres of support, except the informal support. Siblings, especially males, play a major role in all kinds of emotional support followed by parents and secondary kin. Parents, except in their old age, are involved largely in providing financial support and also assist their dependent and non-dependent children. Further, it was also found that friends and siblings of the same age are the largest support to the widows. But if the widows are in the middle age or aged, the parents of most of them may not be alive or even if they were, they were old and lack in economic resources.

Social support speaks about the support that is accessible to people through their social networks. Social networks refer to the structural characteristics of an individual's social relationships, including characteristics of the network, frequency of contact and individual satisfaction with their social contacts. David et al. (2008), while studying the informal social support and older persons' psychological well-being in Hong Kong, observed that the living arrangements of the older persons have the potential to impact the quality and quantity of social support. The effects of size of social network on psychological well-being were stronger for older persons who lived alone than for those who lived with a spouse or relatives. Further, their study also shows that satisfaction with support provided by family members was singled out as the most important correlate of psychological well-being. In other words, the role of family members contributes far more importantly to the well-being compared to other social network members.

Lalitha and Jamuna's (2004) study on widows and widowers in Andhra Pradesh found that widows used more emotion focused coping strategy whereas widowers used slightly more problem focused coping. The less frequently used strategy by both groups was cognitive coping. Further, they found that well-adjusted widows and widowers used problem-focused coping strategy more than emotion-focused and cognitive strategy.

Nasreen (2007), in a study of coping with economic problems in old age and civil society's response, reported that most of the elderly experience financial problems during their old age and most of them want to keep their expenditure within their available resources. They are unable to satisfy even the most basic needs of life for which they have to depend on their children. The situation is more pathetic in the case of elderly widows as many widows do not work even before their widowhood.

Gender-related differences show that women worldwide live longer than men, leading to a process called the 'feminization of later life'. In Hindu society, widowhood is a social death for a woman. The loss of status at the death of husband increases the situation of dependency. This dependency become more as a woman grow older, given the situation that she has no source of income or right to property, where her relationship with her sons and daughters-in-law decides her status in old age. Every phase of widowhood is hard, challenging and deranging and also brings severe social, economic, emotional and cultural deprivation than the widowhood itself (Kumari and Sekher, 2012).

Organization of the Chapters

Chapter 1 (Introduction and Review of Literature) contains introduction to the research theme and review of available literature on elderly widows. Chapter 2 (Objectives, Data Sources and Methodology) gives the description about the significance of the study, objectives, secondary sources of data used for analysis, primary data collection procedure, description about the study area, sampling procedure, and description of analytical techniques used. Chapter 3 (Status of Elderly Widows in India: Secondary Data Analysis) analyse the status of the elderly widows using the available secondary data from various rounds of NSSO and Census of India. Chapter 4 (Profiles of Surveyed Households and Elderly Widows) provides the profile of the elderly widow respondents and their households. A brief description about the selected study villages is also given here. Chapter 5 (Living Arrangements and Economic Status of Elderly Widows) discusses the living arrangements, economic status and dependency levels of the elderly widows. Chapter 6 (Health Status and Treatment Seeking Behaviour of Elderly Widows) analyses the health status and treatment seeking behaviour of elderly widows. Chapter 7 (Vulnerability, Coping Mechanism and Support for Elderly Widows) examines the psycho-social problems, the coping mechanism and the social support available to the surveyed elderly widows. Chapter 8 (Summary, Conclusions and Recommendations) provides the summary, conclusions and policy recommendations emerging from the study.

2

Objectives, Data Sources and Methodology

Significance of the Study

In India, the implications of ageing and our understanding of this process and its impact are still limited. Most of the studies were based on homogeneous group of elderly people, by overlooking the disparities in the experiences in ageing for men and women. Implications of ageing on the lives of elderly are often taken as natural but there are significant differences in the way ageing affects men and women. A major concern relates to the increasing proportion of elderly women, especially widows, in India's population.

The importance of the study on widowhood emerges from the fact that the death of one's spouse precipitates a period of crisis. It brings about a number of economic and social consequences both for the individual and for the family. Widowhood is a turning point in a woman's life, involving new social adjustments for the family as well as for her. Indian women who are widowed are widely discriminated against and seldom receive respect and care from people in general and from the family in particular. Widows have to face many forms of deprivation – economic, social, cultural and emotional. The marital dissolution of the aged persons has a strong bearing on their socio-economic as well as mental well-being. Married persons tend to enjoy higher levels of survival, mental health, social participation and life satisfaction compared to older persons who were widowed. The loss of a companion also leads to weakening of families and social networks, loss of economic power and loss of identity. So, these individuals constitute a special group in our population because of the deprivation, vulnerability and low social status. India is perhaps the only country where widowhood, in addition to being a personal status, exists as a social institution. Widows' deprivation and stigmatization are exacerbated by rituals and religious symbolism. Indian society, similar to all patriarchal societies, confers social status on a woman through a man. Hence, in the absence of a man, she herself becomes a non-entity, ultimately suffering a social death.

The National Policy for Older Persons (Government of India, 1999) assures elderly that their concerns are national concerns and they will not live unprotected, ignored or marginalized. The policy aims to strengthen their legitimate place in society and help older persons to live their last phase of life with purpose, dignity and peace. However, the need and requirement of widows have not been given any priority in the welfare policies. Being a widow and being aged places a woman in a 'double jeopardy' (Prakash, 2000).

The increase in the incidence of widowhood for women as they move up in age requires due consideration as it has implications for financial, emotional and social security (Shankardass, 2003). Study by Folta and Deck (1987) among the Black elderly widows in rural Zimbabwe found that factors such as migration of sons and daughters for employment and desire of the young to establish independent households have contributed to the breakdown in tradition, especially related to inheritance, respect of the elderly and also a sense of responsibility for their well-being. In this context, widows have to suffer since their property is often confiscated by their husband's family and they are left in a situation leading to 'destitution, insecurity and low self-esteem'.

If widowhood is such a neglected social issue, it is partly because the vulnerability associated with losing one's spouse is, overwhelmingly a woman's experience (Dreze and Sen, 2002). Further, the consequences of losing one's spouse are very different for men and women. A widower not only has much greater freedom to remarry than his female counterpart, he also has more extensive property rights, wider opportunities for remunerative employment, and a more authoritative claim on economic support from his children. There are intimate links between the predicament of widows and a wide range of patriarchal institutions in India such as patrilineal inheritance, patrilocal residence and the gender division of labour (Chen and Dreze, 1995).

There is a need to examine the situation of the elderly widows and their economic conditions and social status. The problems that elderly women face are moreover frequently compounded by their difficulties in obtaining sufficient income because of their limited rights to property. Special attention is needed to provide support and care for elderly widows. However, there is a serious dearth of data on social and economic conditions of widows and their health related issues (Chen and Dreze, 1992).

In a number of demographic studies, marital union and determinants of age at marriage have been given more attention as they have implication on fertility. But, not enough attention has been given to study the marital dissolution, and further the status and problems of the widowed.

Most of the widows in rural India are subject to economic hardships, social isolation and related deprivation. They face restrictions on mobility, social participation, inheritance, employment and the kind of social support they receive from relatives and the community. Davis and Blake (1956) highlighted the importance of widowhood as an important intermediate variable affecting fertility. Very few studies have focused on widows as a distinct social group and practically none have attempted to provide a comprehensive analysis of their social and economic conditions. However, widowhood has been an explicit or implicit theme in a number of studies dealing with issues such as old age, living arrangements of the elderly, female-headed households, remarriage practices, etc. Further, studying socio-economic and demographic characteristics of elderly widows in rural set-up will unfold many unexplored issues. Given this background, the proposed study will try to examine few important aspects about the elderly widows:

- What are the problems of the elderly widows?
- To what extent elderly widows are economically dependent?
- Whether widows face discrimination, socially and culturally?

Widowed women have higher rates of physical morbidity, lower levels of life satisfaction, and less social support. They are higher on psychological distress compared to widowers of similar age and are likely to be socially, economically and psychologically marginalized (Sheoran et al., 2004). Existence of stigmatized social perception, negative attitude towards widowhood and lack of social support systems would manifest in poor mental health and problems of adjustment which will make them more vulnerable. Combined effects of ageing and widowhood aggravate the miseries of women in rural areas. Consequently, they experience more social, economic, health and psychological problems in later years of life.

The death of a spouse in old age is known to have profound effects on the well-being of the widow/widower, and is an event which provokes important life changes (Momtaz et al., 2009). This is because older persons may already have a chronic physical illness that decreases their ability to adjust with the bereavement are more likely to become physically ill after the death of a spouse and also may suffer many losses, including financial security. The circumstances of widows vary a great deal between different regions, communities, classes and age groups. Census of India (2001) shows there are more than 19 million elderly widows, comprising about 51 per cent of the total elderly female population of the country. Despite this, little is known about the actual living conditions of elderly widows and the deprivations they experience on a daily basis. Therefore, there is a need to understand the socio-economic and demographic situation of the rural elderly widows. In this context, the present study is an attempt to understand the various aspects related to elderly widows.

The operational definition of 'elderly widows' for the present study includes all widows aged 60 years and above. Age 60 years and above is chosen after recognizing the particular difficulties, like health problems, social problems, economic problems and emotional problems, faced by widows not only because of widowhood but also because of advanced age.

Objectives of the Study

This study is examining the influences of socio-economic and demographic attributes on the status of elderly widows with special emphasis on following aspects – living arrangements, economic dependency, health status, and coping mechanism.

The study has the following specific objectives:

- To examine the living arrangements of elderly widows in rural areas.
- To study the socio-economic status and level of dependency of elderly widows.
- To study the health status (physical and psychological) and the treatment seeking behaviour of elderly widows.
- To understand the extent of vulnerability and the coping mechanism of elderly widows within the family and in the community.

Conceptual Framework

A conceptual framework has been developed to study the direct and indirect impact of the socio-economic and other factors on the well-being of elderly widows. This framework shows the pathways through which the status/well-being/vulnerability of the elderly widows could be determined. It indicates that individual/household characteristics as well as economic and social factors have direct effect on the living arrangement, economic conditions and health status of elderly widows in India. The extent of vulnerability is threefold – they are women, they are widows, and they are aged. The economic position after widowhood affects the living arrangements as well as the health status. Health status in turn will affect the economic status. Finally, all these (living arrangements, economic conditions and health status) variables have impact on the overall status/well-being of the elderly widows. In lieu of these factors, the status of the elderly widows can be analysed by using the framework given in Figure 2.1.

Figure 2.1

Conceptual Framework

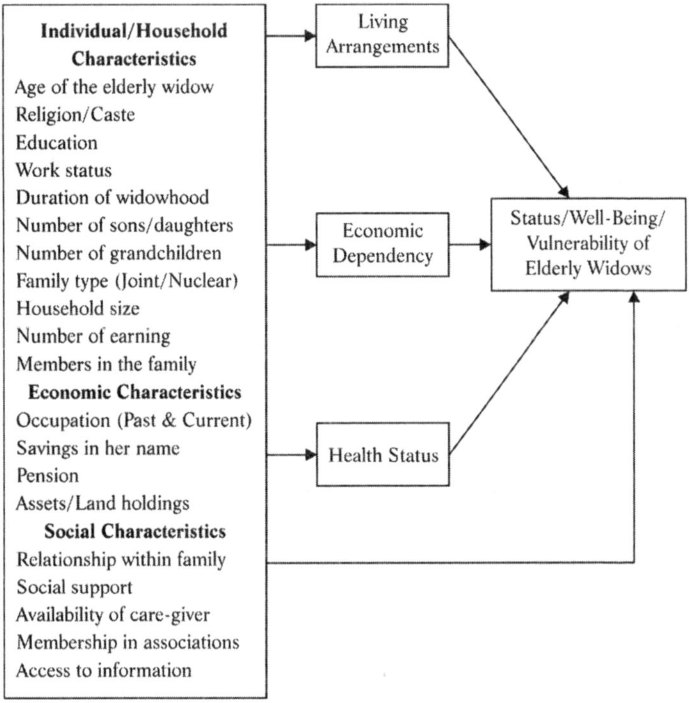

Data Sources and Methodology

In this section, a discussion on the sources of data used in the study, study area, procedure for sample selection and development of survey instruments have been included. The present study has both qualitative and quantitative components. The qualitative data was used to explore issues related to the dependency level of the widows, their relationship with children and other relatives, coping mechanism, the extent and nature of deprivation, etc. To measure the psychological health/well-being, appropriate scales have been used.

Data Sources

In order to understand the social, psychological, economic and other implications on elderly widows, one cannot entirely rely only on available secondary data. So, for the present study both secondary and primary data have been used. NSSO 52nd (1998) and NSSO 60th Rounds (2006) provide information on elderly as well as for elderly widows. A survey of elderly widows has been carried out in the selected villages from two blocks of East Singhbhum district, by using a semi-structured interview schedule.

Secondary Data Sources

(a) Census of India

In order to understand the emerging socio-economic and demographic scenario of elderly and elderly widows in India, the present study utilized the information from various censuses about the age-sex distribution of population, work participation by age groups, disability among the elderly and widows, etc.

(b) National Sample Survey Organization (NSSO)

The National Sample Survey Organization provides information about the elderly persons as well as about the elderly widows in three rounds – 42nd Round (1986–87), 52nd Round (1998) and 60th Round (2006). The data from two rounds of NSSO (52nd and 60th) have been used to examine the status of elderly widows at the national level. The 52nd Round of NSSO primarily focused on health care and education including problems of the aged persons (60 years and above) in India. The total elderly population covered in 52nd Round of NSSO is 33,982 and among them 9,806 are widows. The information was collected on number of living children, living arrangement, economic dependency, number of dependents, state of physical health, disability and familial roles in the household. In the 60th Round of NSSO, in addition to the questions related to the utilization of the health care services and morbidity profile of the population, problems of the aged persons such as economic dependency, living arrangement, support mechanism, physical immobility, etc. are also provided separately. A sample of 34,831 elderly were interviewed (among them 13,287 were widowed) in the 60th Round.

Primary Data Source

The secondary data sets have been analysed to understand the scenario of elderly and elderly widows at the national level.

However, the major analysis of the present study is based on the primary survey which is required to examine the stated objectives. For the purpose of the study, the data have been collected from 300 elderly widows from the two blocks, namely Bahragorda and Ghatshila of East Singhbhum district of Jharkhand state. The interviews were conducted with scientifically designed and pre-tested semi-structured interview schedule, covering issues like – living arrangements, economic conditions, level of dependency, health status, treatment seeking behaviour, and coping mechanism within the family and in the community.

Methods Used for Data Collection

Quantitative Methods

For collecting the quantitative data from the identified households having elderly widows, pre-tested, semi-structured interview schedules were used. Two different sets of interview schedules, namely household schedule and individual schedule, were administered. The individual interview schedule has five broad sections. In the first section, background characteristics of the respondent, relationship with their children, age at widowhood, causes of death of the husband, etc. were included. Section two includes the information about the actual living arrangements, preferred living arrangements, economic condition, perception about the support from children, pension, ownership of land and property, etc. In the third section, health status, treatment seeking behaviour and health adjustment inventory scale for the elderly were included. In the fourth section, information on the social support and coping mechanisms of the elderly widows were covered. The last section provides information about the mistreatment and abuse experienced by the elderly widows within the family and outside the family. In order to understand the psychological condition of elderly widows, geriatric depression scale (GDS) was employed, along with the self-adjustment inventory and social-adjustment inventory for elderly. The interview schedule has both open ended and close ended questions in local language. The data was collected by the researcher with the help of trained female investigators, who were familiar with the area and also had proficiency in local language.

Qualitative Methods

In order to have a deep insight into the problems, it was decided to collect information, which is not available in the interview schedule. Ten case studies of elderly widows have been undertaken from the study villages. Wherever possible, key informant interviews of officials, local leaders, NGOs, doctors were also undertaken.

Selection of Study Area

Jharkhand state is selected for conducting the primary survey. According to 2001 Census, the proportion of elderly is 5.9 per cent in Jharkhand. The sex ratio of elderly (60+ years) is 1,005 females per 1,000 males compared to 941 females to 1,000 males in the general population. All districts of Jharkhand state were ranked according to the proportion of elderly widows. The district having higher proportion of elderly widows, East Singhbhum (7.8%), has been selected for the field study. This district also has highest literacy rate (69.42) in the state, but lowest in female work participation (20.02).

Map 2.1

Map of Jharkhand State

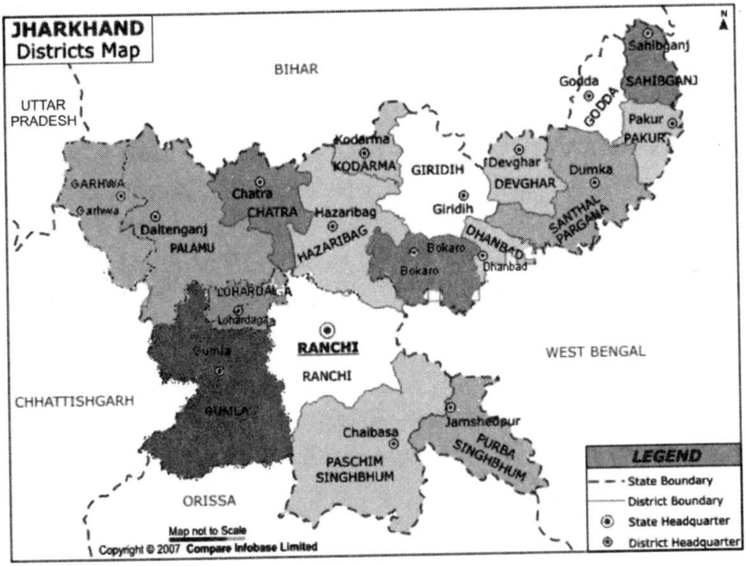

Source: Indiamapstore.com

Before starting the survey, a preliminary visit to the study area was made. From the selected district, two blocks – Bahragorda and Ghatshila – were randomly selected. In Bahragorda block, there are 27 panchayats. Bahragorda panchayat which is having large number of villages (20 villages) was selected for survey. In Jharkhand, the average village size is not very big. So the villages having more than 100 households were selected for the survey. Out of these 20 villages, seven villages were covered in the survey by keeping in mind the availability and accessibility of villages. In Ghatshila block, there are 14 panchayats. One panchayat, namely Kakrisole, was chosen for conducting the survey. Total five villages were covered to collect information from 150 elderly widows from this block. In order to complete the targeted sample size of 300 elderly widows, 12 villages from the two blocks were visited.

Map 2.2

Map of the District and Surveyed Blocks – East Singhbhum

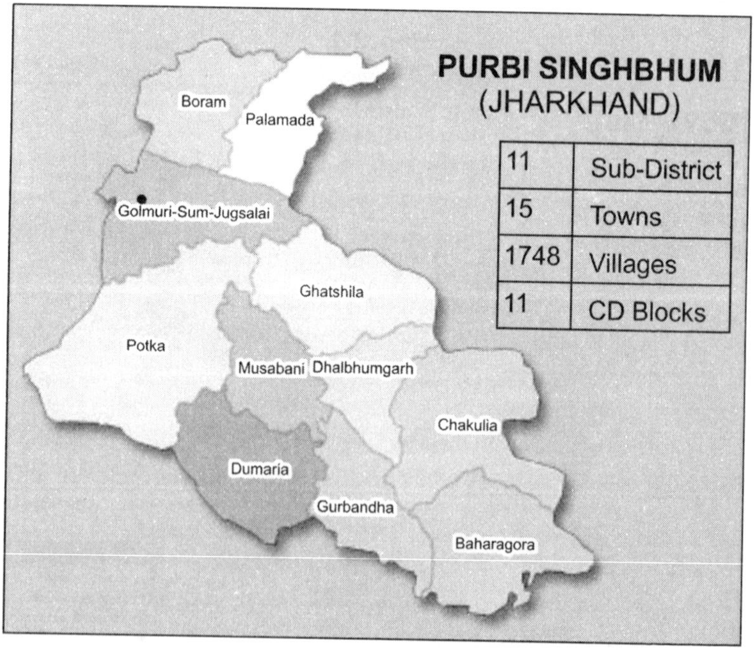

Source: Indiamapstore.com

Sample Selection Procedures

The information was collected from the elderly widows in rural areas of two blocks of the selected district. Three stage sampling design was adopted with the selection of blocks in the first stage, villages in the second stage and households in the third stage. The aim of the study is not to estimate any indicator, but to present and understand the condition of elderly widows of rural areas. So, keeping the time, cost and labour in consideration, it was decided to interview 300 respondents from two blocks, with equal number of respondents from each block. With the help of Anganwadi workers and other locals from the villages, the households with eligible respondents were identified. While conducting the face-to-face interview, respondents were also asked whether they knew any other widow (60 years and above) in their vicinity.

Statistical Methods for Data Analysis

Appropriate univariate and bi-variate analysis have been used. Along with the descriptive statistics such as frequency distribution, mean and median, chi-square test and paired t-test were also applied to understand the existing differentials across various parameters.

Description about Scales Used in the Analysis

Geriatric Depression Scale (GDS): In order to understand the psychological condition or depression level among elderly widows, 'Geriatric Depression Scale' (GDS) was employed. The Geriatric Depression Scale (GDS) was first developed by Yesavage et al. (1983). Dong et al. (2008) found that GDS is an effective scale for assessing depression in community-based studies. GDS consists of 30-item questionnaire in which participants are asked to respond by answering 'yes' or 'no' in reference to how they feel over the past one month. In order to adapt the scale to the Indian situation, certain questions were excluded from the scale as it may not be relevant in Indian context. Certain questions were modified as per the requirement and the scale was finalized. For the purpose of the present study, 24 items have been considered in the scale. Reliability test has been conducted. One point is given for each positive response to the question and by totalling the points counted for each answer, the score of 0–8 shows *'no depression'* or *'normal'*; score of 9–17 indicating *'mild depression'* and score over 18 shows *'severe depression'*.

Adjustment Inventory for the Elderly: The Adjustment Inventory was constructed by Bell (1934) and further it was standardized for Indian situation by Ramamurthy (1968). The original scale consists of 66 items which is known as 'well-adjustment scale'. On the theoretical basis, these 66 items have been grouped into different sub-scales namely, family adjustment, self-adjustment, social-adjustment, emotional adjustment and health adjustment. Health adjustment inventory, self-adjustment inventory and social adjustment inventory for the elderly have been used in the present study.

The health adjustment inventory has 14 items; self-adjustment and social adjustment inventory has 20 items each. Reliability test has been conducted and three different composite indices have been developed. Details about the scale and the scores categorization have been given in the respective chapters where it has been analysed.

Ethical Considerations and Informed Consent

Respect for the elderly has always been a common heritage of mankind (Fenech, 2003). Informed consent from the participants has been taken prior to the interview. Participation was voluntary and the respondent had full liberty to choose not to answer any question or leave the interview at any moment if she felt like. To the extent possible, privacy was maintained at the time of interview. The respondents were given assurance about the confidentiality of the information collected.

Duration of Fieldwork

The data collection was carried out from March to June 2010 in the selected villages of the district of East Singhbhum in Jharkhand state.

Fieldwork Experiences

It was a great learning experience for me to meet and to conduct interviews of elderly widows in the study villages. It was also a challenging task to collect information from the elderly. Before starting the fieldwork, the purpose of the research and survey was explained to the *mukhaiya* (head) of each village. This helped in ensuring co-operation from the villagers. Some of the respondents were curious to know whether they will get any financial benefits from the government. Most of the respondents were willing to share their views and experiences. Some of the elderly widows started weeping while describing their widowhood experiences. Few were hesitant to share their feelings to an 'outsider' like me. Some interviews could be completed only after two or three sittings.

Visiting the Villages

Before starting the fieldwork, I made a preliminary visit of the selected blocks. First I met the headman of the village and explained the purpose of my survey. Initially, some were not convinced about my intention. Several times they asked me – 'what benefits will we get out of your survey?' Some of them thought that I am from a government department and wanted to know the situation of the old people in that area. I also met the Block Development Officers (BDO) and sought their co-operation.

Meeting with Respondents

The first field visit was made with the help of village headman. He introduced me to one house where an elderly widow was staying. I introduced myself and explained my purpose of visit. She was not ready to talk to me as her son was not at home and asked me to come on another day. After requesting her again she get ready for the interview. We started with a general talk. She answered all my questions. Since this was my first day and first interview, it took almost three hours to complete the interview.

When I finished the interview, she said – 'One more elderly widow is staying near to my house, if you want I can take you to her house'. She took me and introduced me to that woman. The elderly widows were very co-operative but the first question from many elderly widows was – 'Are you from the pension department?' Few of them, who were not receiving the pension, said – 'Please get my pension sanctioned. I have visited the Block Office several times, but they keep saying that I am not old enough to get the pension'. This shows the helpless situation of elderly widows in many villages and their difficulty in getting any assistance from the government. Some of them were very happy to share their feelings and concerns with me. Some of them offered tea and lunch during interviews and asked me to visit their houses again.

3

Status of Elderly Widows in India

Secondary Data Analysis

Ageing Scenario and Status of Elderly Widows in India

The aged population in India records a gradual 'feminization' and serious gender disparities. The feminization of ageing is evident from the growth pattern of the elderly females which remained varying over the past decades (Alam, 2006). It was earlier considered that population ageing was a problem of only developed countries. But the recent trends show that it is increasing rapidly in developing countries, including India. Figure 3.1 shows that in 2001 the proportion of elderly in India was 7.5 per cent which is likely to increase at much faster pace in coming decades. The proportion of female elderly is higher than that of the male elderly in India. The increasing proportion of elderly women, especially widows, in the population is a major concern.

The marital status of the elderly assumes special significance in the context of care in old age. According to 2001 Census, 33 per cent of the elderly in India lived without spouses. Of the male elderly, 15 per cent were widowers. Among female elderly, 51 per cent are widows. The proportion of widows is much higher as compared to the widowers; a characteristic feature of India's aged population.

Age, sex and marital status are important demographic characteristics of any population. In India, depending upon the marital status of the elderly, especially that of women, their position and status within the family as well as in the society will be determined. From Table 3.1, it can be easily seen that widows are outnumbering widowers. The distribution of population by their marital status shows that a higher proportion of elderly women are widows.

Figure 3.1

Proportion of Aged (60 years and above) in India, 2001

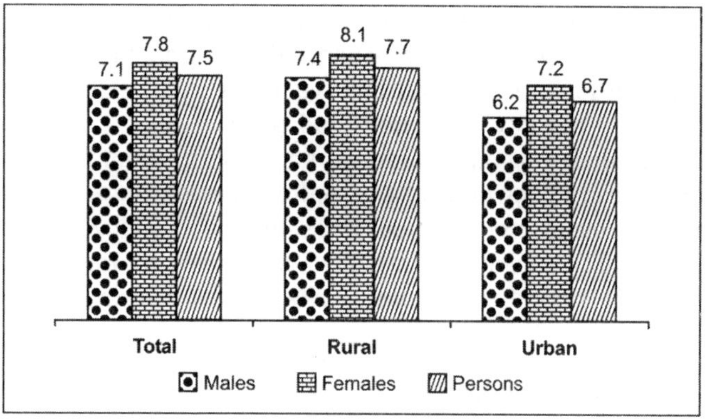

Source: Census of India, 2001.

Table 3.1

*India's Elderly Population by Age, Sex and Marital Status, 2001**

Age	*Sex*	*Marital Status*				*Total*
		NM	*M*	*W*	*D/S*	
60+ Years	Males	2.5	82.1	15.0	0.3	49.3
	Females	1.5	47.3	50.7	0.5	50.7
60–64	Males	1.9	88.0	9.8	0.3	49.4
	Females	1.1	58.3	40.0	0.6	50.6
65–69	Males	2.1	85.1	12.5	0.3	47.8
	Females	1.2	53.4	45.0	0.5	52.2
70–79	Males	2.8	78.3	18.6	0.3	50.8
	Females	1.6	35.5	62.5	0.4	49.2
80+ Years	Males	5.4	65.3	28.9	0.4	48.8
	Females	3.5	25.1	71.0	0.4	51.2

Note: NM: Never Married, M: Married, W: Widowed, D/S: Divorced/Separated.

* India conducted the latest census in 2011. However, the data on age structure of the population is yet to be released.

Source: Census of India (2001).

In India, the prevalence of widowhood is higher than widowerhood. Table 3.2 indicates that the age-specific prevalence of widowhood among men is low compared to that of women. The age-specific prevalence of widowhood has decreased over the decades. The proportion of widows in the female population rises sharply with age, reaching well over half among women (aged 60 years and above) and more than two-thirds among women aged 70 years and above. Thus, the Indian woman who survives to old age is most likely to become a widow (Dreze and Sen, 2002). The high incidence of widowhood could be one of the important factors responsible for the lower status and high vulnerability of elderly women. Widowers do not face restrictions and social stigma. In most cases, they retain their economic resources and have freedom for mobility. However, restrictions on mobility and association make it hard for women to overcome isolation once they are widowed (United Nations, 2002). Older men usually have wives to care for them whereas that is not the case for majority of older women in India.

Table 3.2

Age and Sex Specific Prevalence of Widowhood in India, 1961–2001 (%)

Age Group	*Prevalence of Widowhood in India*									
	Males					*Females*				
	1961	*1971*	*1981*	*1991*	*2001*	*1961*	*1971*	*1981*	*1991*	*2001*
10–14	0.07	0.04	0.02	0.04	0.04	0.13	0.05	0.03	0.06	0.13
15–19	0.29	0.02	0.09	0.07	0.06	0.52	0.34	0.21	0.18	0.20
20–24	0.90	0.58	0.38	0.31	0.24	1.29	0.88	0.69	0.59	0.68
25–29	1.67	1.25	0.78	0.61	0.55	2.89	1.94	1.50	1.15	1.37
32–34	2.67	1.99	1.34	1.01	0.90	6.42	4.09	3.12	2.32	2.59
35–39	3.67	2.66	1.94	1.32	1.24	11.14	7.04	5.42	3.94	4.45
42–44	5.98	4.43	3.31	2.32	1.85	20.66	14.38	10.86	7.71	7.71
45–49	8.24	5.90	4.46	3.17	2.57	28.84	20.66	15.96	11.16	11.31
50–54	12.37	9.64	7.34	5.58	4.35	45.47	36.60	29.71	21.93	20.18
55–59	15.53	12.07	8.97	6.85	5.93	50.24	41.22	31.79	23.76	21.95
60–64	21.83	17.15	14.11	11.16	9.83	69.62	62.41	56.05	45.24	40.00
65–69	25.87	20.41	17.21	13.39	12.46	71.84	64.59	58.55	48.10	44.92
70+	36.10	30.45	27.04	21.39	21.36	84.38	80.36	77.55	67.20	64.87

Source: Census of India (various years).

While examining this phenomenon, it can be seen that gap in the widowhood proportion gets bridged up among the old-old (70+ years). In 2001, 65 per cent of the old-old women are widows whereas only 21 per cent of the old-old men are widowers. In Indian context, widowhood means a loss of self-esteem, dignity, social position and rights. Widows are the unfortunate victims of nature and for centuries they have been ill-treated (Pandya and Shah, 2006). Widows have to face many forms of deprivation – economic, social, cultural and emotional. Widowhood of aged persons has a strong bearing on their socio-economic as well as mental well-being. So, these individuals constitute a special group in our population because of deprivation, vulnerability and low social status. Widows have to face increased economic problems after the death of the husband. It is generally believed that the elderly are a burden to the family and they do not contribute to the national income (Siva Raju, 2011). They are forced to work in order to earn a living. In India, 40 per cent of the elderly who are 60 years and above are still working (Bhagat and Unisa, 2006).

Since census does not give information about the work participation according to the marital status, so a general view of the work participation among the elderly has been analysed. It can be seen from Table 3.3 that the work participation rate among males of aged 60 years and above are three times higher than that of females of same age.

Table 3.3

Work Participation by Age and Sex in India and Jharkhand, 2001

Age Group	*India*			*Jharkhand*		
	Persons	*Males*	*Females*	*Persons*	*Males*	*Females*
All age groups	39.1	51.7	25.6	37.5	48.0	26.4
15–59 years	61.1	80.7	40.0	61.8	78.8	43.5
60+ years	40.3	60.3	20.9	41.4	60.9	22.1

Source: Census of India and Jharkhand, 2001.

According to 2001 Census, a 'main worker' is the one who had participated in any economically productive activity for a period of more than six months, at any time during the reference period of preceding one year. A person who had worked for less than six months during the reference period was defined as 'marginal worker'. 'Work' included even part-time help or unpaid work on farm, family enterprise or in any other economic activity. A person who did not work at all during the reference period was considered as 'non-worker'. In India, more than 80 per cent males aged 60 years and above are working as main workers whereas only 57 per cent of females aged 60 years and above are engaged in main work (Table 3.4).

Table 3.4

Work Participation as Main Workers and Marginal Workers by Age and Sex, in India and Jharkhand, 2001

Age Group	*India*					
	Main Workers			*Marginal Workers*		
	Persons	*Males*	*Females*	*Persons*	*Males*	*Females*
All age groups	30.4	45.1	14.7	22.2	12.7	42.7
15–59 years	78.8	88.3	58.3	21.2	11.7	41.7
60+ years	79.7	87.7	57.3	20.3	12.3	42.7

Source: Census of India, 2001

Aged women who lose their spouse are often forced to leave households, move with children or relatives and give up claims on property. Widows have an inferior status compared to widowers and the majority is poor and economically dependent. Since most of the family assets are acquired in the name of the man, the widow, unemployed or under employed without any savings for old age, ultimately ends up in dependency and misery during her old age. One of the social security pension schemes for poor widows is the Destitute Old and Widow's Pension Scheme, which makes old dependents less of a burden for their families (Jamuna, 2008). Widowhood is the major factor which influences one's adjustment and mental health. In this chapter, an attempt was made to analyse the status of the elderly widows by using available secondary data.

Socio-Economic and Demographic Characteristics of Elderly Widows in India

Table 3.5 shows the socio-economic and demographic characteristics of widowed in India. More than half of the widows are in the age group of 60–69, and one-fourth (31%) are in old-old (70–79) age group, 85 per cent of the widows are illiterate compared to 57 per cent of the all elderly. Less than 2 per cent of elderly widows have education up to secondary level and above. More than three-fourth of the widow population lives in rural areas. It can be also observed that majority of the elderly widows are engaged in unpaid family work. Only 9 per cent of them are getting pension or remittances compared to 12 per cent of all elderly.

In India, it is traditionally believed that a son will take care of parents in their old age while daughters leave the house after marriage. The number of sons in a household could be a crucial determinant in overall status of the elderly respondent's life.

Seven per cent of the widows have reported that they do not have any son whereas less than one-tenth of the widows have reported having no daughters.

Table 3.5

Socio-Economic and Demographic Characteristics of Elderly Widows and Aged in India (% distribution)

Socio-Economic and Demographic Characteristics	*Elderly Widows*	*Elderly Widowers*	*Elderly Females*	*All Elderly*
Age group				
Young-old (60–69 years)	56.9	48.7	79.7	71.9
Old-old (70–79 years)	31.4	32.0	17.1	22.7
Oldest-old (80+ years)	11.7	19.3	3.1	5.5
Place of residence				
Rural	75.2	79.8	75.1	75.4
Urban	24.8	20.2	24.9	24.6
Religion				
Hindu	84.3	86.3	84.0	84.0
Muslim	10.1	8.4	8.0	9.0
Christian	2.7	2.0	3.2	2.8
Others	2.9	3.3	4.8	4.2

Cont'd...

...Cont'd

Caste				
SC	17.7	18.2	16.6	17.2
ST	7.0	7.7	5.7	6.2
OBC	40.8	42.2	39.0	39.0
Others	34.6	31.9	38.7	37.6
Educational level				
Not literate	85.2	62.3	75.5	56.8
Below primary level	6.4	13.3	7.5	12.1
Below secondary level	6.7	17.5	11.3	18.5
Secondary level and above	1.8	6.9	5.7	12.5
Usual activity status				
Self-employed	4.7	25.7	2.2	27.4
Regular employment	0.6	1.0	0.3	1.7
Casual labour/Daily wage earner	5.4	7.0	5.3	9.5
Unpaid family worker*	35.6	7.4	68.5	25.5
Pensioners/Remittance receivers	9.1	12.7	3.7	11.8
Others	44.6	46.3	20.0	24.1
Number of sons				
No son	7.1	5.0	5.0	4.9
One son	30.9	25.9	25.4	25.9
Two sons	28.8	31.3	32.5	33.7
Three sons	18.8	24.2	20.7	20.3
More than three sons	14.4	13.6	16.4	15.3
Number of daughters				
No daughter	9.2	8.6	6.8	7.1
One daughter	32.8	34.8	29.2	30.7
Two daughters	29.0	28.7	29.9	30.2
Three daughters	16.6	17.6	19.0	17.8
More than three daughters	12.4	10.3	15.1	14.2
Total Respondents	**10,011**	**3,267**	**7,070**	**21,553**

Note: Elderly females (all aged women other than widows), all elderly (all aged men and women excluding widows and widowers).

* worked as helper in household enterprise/farm, etc.

Source: NSSO 60th Round (2006).

Living Arrangements of Elderly Widows in India

The living arrangement is an important component of the welfare of aged population. Since the elderly are less able to remain

Table 3.6

Living Arrangements of Elderly Widows and Aged in India

Living Arrangements	*Rural*				*Urban*			
	Elderly Widows	*Elderly Widowers*	*Elderly Females*	*All Elderly*	*Elderly Widows*	*Elderly Widowers*	*Elderly Females*	*All Elderly*
Living alone*	12.4	10.3	1.4	1.1	10.3	7.4	0.9	1.1
Living with spouse only	NA	NA	21.1	20.3	NA	NA	18.4	16.7
Living with spouse and others	NA	NA	68.2	70.8	NA	NA	71.4	74.1
Living without spouse but with children	74.5	81.7	5.9	4.1	75.4	83.7	5.6	4.6
Living with other relations and non-relations	12.7	7.0	3.4	3.6	14.1	7.1	3.8	3.6
Total Respondents	6,206	2,199	4,531	13,809	3,805	997	2,539	7,744

Note: Elderly females (all aged women other than widows), all elderly (all aged men and women excluding widows and widowers).

* Living alone includes: living as an inmate of old age home as well as not as an inmate of old age home.

Source: NSSO 60th Round (2006).

independent, they need care and support of others in several respects. Living arrangements are usually influenced by variety of factors such as number and availability of children and other relatives, kinship patterns of the society, location of household, financial status, and also availability of support services. Further, attitudes towards and perceptions about the living place are other important factors that decide where one prefers to live (Chen, 1998). Living arrangements of the elderly widows and the aged in India is presented in Table 3.6. As expected, most of the elderly widows (75%) are living with their children, illustrating the fact that family is still the major care-taker for the aged in India. However, about 12 per cent of elderly widows in rural areas are living alone compared to only 1 per cent of the aged in rural areas. This is a clear indication of lack of family support, persisting gender discrimination and increasing vulnerability of widows.

Economic Dependency and Persons Financially Supporting Elderly Widows

An important factor that affects the status of widows and especially elderly widows are economic viability. A widowed woman's life could be highly disrupted if she does not have economic means of support. If elderly women have an adequate income, it largely meets their material needs and comforts. Dependency is one of the reasons for elderly to continue to work in their old age, in spite of poor health (Rajan and Prasad, 2008).

High level of economic dependency is one of the major problems faced by elderly widows. The National Sample Survey also provides information regarding the economic dependency of the elderly. All elderly were asked to describe the state of their economic dependency and their responses were grouped into three categories – *not dependent, partially dependent,* and *fully dependent*. In India, around three-fourth of the rural elderly widows are economically fully dependent on others for their day-to-day maintenance, whereas less than half of the aged are in that category. In urban areas also, the proportion of elderly widows who are economically dependent on others is more compared to the aged population. This illustrates the extent of deprivation of elderly widows (Table 3.7).

The family is the major support for the majority of older persons, especially for elderly widows, and those who have no

Table 3.7

Economic Dependency among Elderly Widows and Aged in India

Dependency Level	*Rural*				*Urban*			
	Elderly Widows	*Elderly Widowers*	*Elderly Females*	*All Elderly*	*Elderly Widows*	*Elderly Widowers*	*Elderly Females*	*All Elderly*
Not dependent	14.0	33.0	29.2	42.2	20.7	38.0	33.9	44.4
Partially dependent	11.4	14.5	16.0	15.7	9.6	14.0	11.0	12.1
Fully dependent	74.5	52.6	54.8	42.1	69.6	48.1	55.1	43.5
Total Respondents	6,206	2,250	4,429	13,509	3,763	1,017	2,489	7,624

Note: Elderly females (all aged women other than widows), all elderly (all aged men and women excluding widows and widowers).
Source: NSSO 60th Round (2006).

Table 3.8

Persons Financially Supporting Elderly Widows and Aged in India

Persons Financially Supporting	*Rural*				*Urban*			
	Elderly Widows	*Elderly Widowers*	*Elderly Females*	*All Elderly*	*Elderly Widows*	*Elderly Widowers*	*Elderly Females*	*All Elderly*
Spouse	NA	NA	24.6	22.2	NA	NA	27.8	24.6
Own children	86.7	88.0	68.4	70.9	85.3	86.8	64.1	68.2
Grandchildren	4.2	3.1	1.5	1.6	4.1	4.6	1.2	1.3
Others	6.8	8.9	5.4	5.2	7.8	8.7	6.9	5.9
Total Number	5,306	1,424	3,117	7,798	3,054	598	1,655	4,163

Note: This is based on the aged and widows who reported that they are dependent on others for economic support.
Elderly females (all aged women other than widows), all elderly (all aged men and women excluding widows and widowers).
Source: NSSO 60th Round (2006).

Table 3.9

Per cent Distribution of Elderly Widows and Aged by Ownership and Management of Property in India

Ownership and Management of Property	*Rural*				*Urban*			
	Elderly Widows	*Elderly Widowers*	*Elderly Females*	*All Elderly*	*Elderly Widows*	*Elderly Widowers*	*Elderly Females*	*All Elderly*
Ownership of the property and managing	16.2	51.6	26.8	54.1	18.7	43.4	23.4	50.7
Ownership but not managing property	24.9	20.3	25.2	17.9	19.7	20.7	24.4	16.2
Not owning but managing property	2.4	2.8	5.3	3.2	2.0	1.4	4.4	3.2
Not owning and not managing property	55.1	22.3	41.1	23.4	57.6	33.1	46.4	28.5

Note: Total may not add to 100 because some have not answered some of the particular questions.
Elderly females (all aged women other than widows), all elderly (all aged men and women excluding widows and widowers).

Source: NSSO 52nd Round (1998).

independent income. Most of the widows in India are financially supported by their own children (Table 3.8). The Indian culture emphasizes the reverential treatment to be given to the aged persons, especially to widows in the family. However, the fast changing family structure from joint families to nuclear ones, has adversely affected the protection and welfare of the aged.

Ownership and Management of Property by Elderly Widows in India

NSSO 52nd Round provides the information about the ownership and management of financial assets of the elderly. The information on the financial assets was taken from two questions regarding the participation by the aged in: (i) ownership and management of financial assets, (ii) ownership and management of property. The responses are categorized into those who have: (a) ownership of the property and managing, (b) ownership but not managing, (c) do not have ownership but managing, (d) neither ownership nor managing the property. The analysis shows that in rural areas, around 54 per cent of the aged have ownership of property and are also managing the property, whereas 55 per cent of the elderly widows in rural areas neither have ownership of property nor are they managing any property (Table 3.9).

In urban areas also, the situation of the elderly widows are the same. Findings also indicate that one-fourth of the widows from rural areas and one-fifth from urban areas are having ownership of property but not managing them. Even those having property are not in a position to manage in a way illustrates their dependency on others and vulnerability.

Basic Unmet Need among Elderly Widows in India

To assess the problems faced by the elderly as well as widows in meeting the basic necessities of life, such as food, clothing and medical care, information was gathered in 52nd Round of the National Sample Survey. All the elderly were asked – *'Are your day-to-day requirements on the following (food, clothes and medicines) adequately met?'* This brought out the dismal situation prevailing in India. In rural areas, 3 per cent of the widows reported difficulty in getting adequate food. The survey indicated that 12 per cent of the widows in rural areas and 6 per cent in

Table 3.10

Basic Unmet Need among Elderly Widows and Aged in India

Unmet Need for	*Rural*				*Urban*			
	Elderly Widows	*Elderly Widowers*	*Elderly Females*	*All Elderly*	*Elderly Widows*	*Elderly Widowers*	*Elderly Females*	*All Elderly*
Food	3.5	2.4	2.5	2.5	2.2	1.0	1.3	1.4
Clothing	5.4	3.9	4.4	3.9	3.3	1.7	1.6	1.8
Medicine	11.7	10.6	8.7	8.4	6.1	3.2	3.6	4.0
At least one	12.0	11.0	9.0	8.7	6.3	3.2	3.8	4.2
All three	3.1	2.0	2.3	2.3	1.9	1.0	1.1	1.1

Note: Elderly females (all aged women other than widows), all elderly (all aged men and women excluding widows and widowers).

Source: NSSO 52nd Round (1998).

Table 3.11

Participation in Social and Religious Activities by Elderly Widows and Aged in India

Participation in	*Rural*				*Urban*			
	Elderly Widows	*Elderly Widowers*	*Elderly Females*	*All Elderly*	*Elderly Widows*	*Elderly Widowers*	*Elderly Females*	*All Elderly*
Social activities	61.5	75.0	76.7	80.9	67.0	73.9	76.6	80.3
Religious activities	71.4	79.3	84.6	84.9	76.8	82.0	87.2	87.1
Total respondents	5,871	2,331	4,333	12,730	3,935	1,046	2,659	8,044

Note: Elderly females (all aged women other than widows), all elderly (all aged men and women excluding widows and widowers).

Source: NSSO 52nd Round (1998).

urban areas faced difficulties in having at least one of the basic needs. About 3 per cent of rural widows and around 2 per cent in urban areas stated that they face difficulties in meeting the requirements for all the three – food, clothing and medicine (Table 3.10). Twelve per cent of rural widows reported unmet need for medicines. Unfortunately, there is no social security measure available to take care of the basic needs of elderly in India. So, the economically poor among the aged, especially widows, have no option but to suffer silently.

Participation in Social and Religious Activities

It is generally felt that a widow's participation in social activities is lower than others. Information on participation in specific activities was also collected in the survey. The elderly were asked: '*Do you participate in social and religious matters?*' Table 3.11 shows that only 62 per cent of rural elderly widows participated in social activities. Participation in religious activities by the urban elderly widows is slightly higher than of their rural counterparts. However, the participation of widows in social as well as religious activities is considerably lower compared to that of other elderly.

Health Status of Elderly Widows in India

The growing number of elderly means that more and more people will be entering the old age when the risk of developing certain chronic and debilitating diseases is significantly higher. The health condition suggests that aged need physical care and support from others who are staying with them. Ageing is a time of multiple illness and general disability. Along with the changes due to old age, life style factors are also contributing disorders and diseases. The NSSO collects information about the most common health problems as reported by the elderly. The extent of diseases reported by the elderly widows is higher than that of the aged. The most reported health problem by elderly widows is the disorder of joints and bones. The cardiovascular disease (hypertension and heart problems) was second highest among the reported diseases (Table 3.12).

Table 3.12

Major Diseases Reported by Elderly Widows and Aged in India

Diseases	*Rural*				*Urban*			
	Elderly Widows	*Elderly Widowers*	*Elderly Females*	*All Elderly*	*Elderly Widows*	*Elderly Widowers*	*Elderly Females*	*All Elderly*
Gastro-intestinal*	2.5	2.0	2.2	2.3	1.2	1.1	1.2	1.3
Cardiovascular	3.5	1.9	3.6	3.5	9.8	7.9	11.1	10.1
Tuberculosis/Bronchial asthma	3.3	4.6	3.0	3.4	2.7	2.7	3.3	3.1
Disorder of joints and bones	8.3	8.2	7.2	6.5	10.3	6.6	7.4	6.4
Diabetes mellitus	1.6	1.0	2.2	2.2	6.4	4.7	7.7	7.5
Total Respondents	6,206	2,250	4,531	13,809	3,805	1,017	2,539	7,744

Note: Elderly females (all aged women other than widows), all elderly (all aged men and women excluding widows and widowers) Information about the major five diseases reported by the respondents has been presented here.

* Gastro-intestinal ailments include diarrhoea/dysentery, gastritis/gastric or peptic ulcer, worm infestation, amoebiosis, hepatitis/jaundice. However, the survey collected information on other diseases, such as neurological disorders, psychiatric disorders, conjunctivitis, glaucoma, etc.

Source: NSSO 60th Round (2006).

Table 3.13

Perception about Current Health Status among Elderly Widows and Aged in India

Health Status	*Rural*				*Urban*			
	Elderly Widows	*Elderly Widowers*	*Elderly Females*	*All Elderly*	*Elderly Widows*	*Elderly Widowers*	*Elderly Females*	*All Elderly*
Excellent	3.4	4.4	3.8	5.7	4.7	5.9	5.6	7.7
Good/Fair	67.2	68.0	72.6	72.8	70.3	69.2	72.8	73.6
Poor	29.4	27.6	23.5	21.5	25.0	24.8	21.6	18.7
Total respondents	5,948	2,133	4,287	13,068	3,673	967	2,410	7,388

Note: Elderly females (all aged women other than widows), all elderly (all aged men and women excluding widows and widowers).

Source: NSSO 60th Round (2006).

Table 3.14

Physical Mobility of Elderly Widows and Aged in India

Mobility Status	*Rural*				*Urban*			
	Elderly Widows	*Elderly Widowers*	*Elderly Females*	*All Elderly*	*Elderly Widows*	*Elderly Widowers*	*Elderly Females*	*All Elderly*
Confined to bed	1.9	1.6	1.5	1.2	2.1	2.7	1.8	1.4
Confined to home	9.2	7.9	5.5	5.0	10.2	9.3	5.6	4.6
Physically mobile	89.0	90.4	93.0	93.8	87.7	88.0	92.6	94.0
Total respondents	6,087	2,195	4,404	1,3431	3,744	996	2,479	7,577

Note: Elderly females (all aged women other than widows), all elderly (all aged men and women excluding widows and widowers).
Source: NSSO 60th Round (2006).

Table 3.15

Disability among Elderly Widows and Aged in India

Disability	*Rural*				*Urban*			
	Elderly Widows	*Elderly Widowers*	*Elderly Females*	*All Elderly*	*Elderly Widows*	*Elderly Widowers*	*Elderly Females*	*All Elderly*
Locomotor disability	44.4	42.4	52.4	51.9	59.2	43.3	61.9	60.6
Visual disability	38.9	39.7	33.8	34.9	27.3	31.4	25.2	27.4
Speech disability	0.3	0.4	0.1	0.2	0.4	0.7	1.0	1.0
Hearing disability	16.4	17.5	13.7	12.9	13.0	24.5	12.0	11.0
Total respondents	1,267	414	711	2,006	734	150	340	928

Note: Elderly females (all aged women other than widows), all elderly (all aged men and women excluding widows and widowers).
Source: NSSO 60th Round (2006).

Perception about Current Health Status among Elderly Widows

The perception about one's own health is an important factor in understanding a person's actual health condition. A person may be considered as being in good health if s/he feels so. Moreover, it reflects the mental health of that person. Very few elderly widows have reported their current health status as excellent or very good in both rural and in urban India. More than one-fifth (29%) of the rural elderly widows perceived their health as poor compared to slightly less than one-fourth of the aged. This is true even in urban areas (Table 3.13).

Physical Mobility of Elderly Widows in India

The ability to move is an indicator of physical condition of a person and the degree of dependence on others for performing daily routine activities. Survey collected information about the physical mobility of the elderly. According to the survey (Table 3.14), more than four-fifth of elderly widows are physically mobile in rural and urban areas. About 2 per cent of them are confined to bed, both in rural and urban areas. Another 10 per cent are confined to home and have difficulty to go outside.

Disability among Elderly Widows in India

Disability and impairments leading to immobility among the elderly is a cause of concern for ageing individuals as it adversely affects their quality of life increasing their risk of dependence and also loss of autonomy (Rajan and Sreerupa, 2008). Regarding the disabilities, about 52 per cent among rural elderly have reported locomotor disability, followed by visual (35%) and hearing disability (13%). This health condition also suggests that the aged need physical care and support from others who are staying with them (Table 3.15). According to Census of India (2001), more elderly widows are disabled as compared to elderly widowers. Three per cent of elderly widows are mentally disabled.

According to Census of India (2001), the visual disability is higher among elderly, much more among female elderly. Around five per cent of aged also reported mental problems This may be much lower than the actual situation (Table 3.16).

Table 3.16

Disability among Elderly (60 years and above) in India

Disability	*Combined*		*Rural*		*Urban*	
	Males	*Females*	*Males*	*Females*	*Males*	*Females*
In vision	49.2	54.7	49.7	55.4	47.2	52.1
In speech	3.3	3.2	3.2	3.1	3.9	3.6
In hearing	11.9	13.3	12.3	13.5	10.1	12.6
In movement	30.8	24.0	30.3	23.7	32.5	25.4
Mental	4.8	4.8	4.5	4.4	6.3	6.3
Disabled	15.6	19.5	16.7	20.9	12.3	15.3

Source: Census of India, 2001.

Social Security and Pension Schemes for Widows and Elderly in India

Social security pensions are basically intended to provide income support to persons adversely affected by events like retrenchment, sickness, physical disability, old age and/or widowhood. In all the states of India, schemes have existed since the early 1960s, addressing the destitute, old and widows. In India, social support for widows differs from state to state.

A quick review of some of the social security or pension schemes and programmes in various states (Prasad, 1998) reveal the following:

(i) Almost all states and Union Territories have Old Age Pension (OAP) and Widows Pension Schemes (WPS). All persons above the age of 65 years are eligible for the OAP, irrespective of gender. Elderly destitute widows are usually considered for pension under the OAP only, though in Kerala young widows are also eligible for this pension.

(ii) Government of India has recently (Government of India, 2009) introduced two schemes for widows and physically disabled i.e. Indira Gandhi National Widow Pension Scheme (IGNWPS) and Indira Gandhi National Disability Pension Scheme (IGNDPS) under National Social Assistance Programme (NSAP). The objective of the IGNWPS is to give financial assistance of ₹ 200 per month to all the identified pensioners who are widows in the age group of 40–64 years, and from families which are below the poverty line. They are eligible to get the pension till she attains the age of 65 years or till her remarriage. The government has also proposed to give priority to young widows (age group 18–40 years) in admission to industrial training institutes (ITI). The Government will bear the expenses of their training and provide them with a monthly stipend of ₹ 500.

Under the IGNDPS, the objective is to provide the financial assistance of ₹ 200 per month to all the identified beneficiaries who are in the age group of 18–64 years, with severe disability (i.e. more than 80% disability) or multiple disability (having more than one disability and at least 40% incapacitation in each type of disability) and from families which are below the poverty line of either sex will be eligible to get the benefit of the scheme.

State Specific Pension Schemes

Tamil Nadu, Gujarat, Odisha and Kerala have pension schemes for destitute widows, whether old or young, and for the physically challenged. Tamil Nadu, Kerala and a few other states extend a one-time assistance to young destitute widows for performing death rites for their deceased husbands or for the marriage of their daughters. Tamil Nadu also has a pension scheme for destitute widows (40 years and above), a similar pension scheme exists in Odisha for destitute widows who are 50 years and above and in Gujarat for widows who are 45 years and above. They are also eligible for the OAP at the age of 65, if they remain destitute. Karnataka has a pension scheme for all widows (18 years and above).

- *Old age and Widow Pension in Maharashtra:* Under the Sanjay Gandhi Niradhar Anudhan Yojana, an individual (females 60 years or above and males 65 years or above) can get ₹ 100 per month, if he/she has no source of income. If a woman is widow and has one or more children below 18 years then she is eligible for a pension of ₹ 250 per month.
- *Widow Pension in West Bengal:* The pension amount is ₹ 150 per month for widows from below poverty line households. There is no age bar.

- *Widow Pension in Kerala*: The pension amount is ₹ 110 per month. The person must be a destitute and her income per year must be below ₹ 12,000. There is no age bar.
- *Widow Pension in Jharkhand:* Under Indira Gandhi National Old Age Pension Scheme (IGNOAPS) persons aged 65 years or above, belonging to BPL category, are entitled to a monthly pension of ₹ 200. Widows in age group 40–64 years are eligible for pension of ₹ 200 per month. The age criterion was revised to 18–64 years for destitute widows.

Summary

The elderly widows constitute one of the most vulnerable groups which need urgent attention. Fifty-one per cent of aged (60 years and above) women in India are widows. An analysis was undertaken using the data from the nationally representative sample survey of NSSO to understand the living arrangements, economic status and health condition of the elderly and widows.

There are several important findings that emerge from this analysis. The elderly widows are economically more dependent than aged population. Most of the widows are living with their children, which indicate that family still play an important role in the living arrangements and welfare of the aged in India. The basic unmet need for food, cloth and medicine is higher among the widows compared to others. Elderly widows' participation in social and religious activities is relatively low compared to the elderly in general. More elderly widows have perceived their health as poor, compared to others among the aged. Widowhood determines the economic status of older women wherein they lack the opportunity to benefit from their spouse's earnings and support.

The ongoing debate on the welfare of the aged in India usually ignores the specific problems of elderly widows and their extent of vulnerability. In the absence of any social security measures, majority of elderly widows continue to live in poverty, ill-health and neglect. The economic dependency compounded by physical and social vulnerability makes them one of the most deprived sections of the Indian society. Social security measures and welfare programmes need to be formulated keeping these factors into consideration.

4

Profiles of Surveyed Households and Elderly Widows

This chapter gives information on the background characteristics of the study population based on the household survey carried out during March to June 2010 in the selected villages of the district of East Singhbhum in Jharkhand state. Drawing data from the household survey, this chapter profiles the surveyed households in terms of their socio-demographic and housing characteristics, including benefits received from the government. The chapter also presents the socio-demographic characteristics of the elderly widows interviewed for the study.

Household Characteristics of the Surveyed Population

The selected characteristics pertaining to the households surveyed are presented in Table 4.1. Distribution by religion suggests that 80 per cent of the surveyed households were Hindus, 13 per cent belonged to the *Sarna** religion and 7 per cent were Muslims 40 per cent of households were Scheduled Tribes, followed by Other Backward Classes (37.3%). Scheduled Castes and general castes comprised 14 and 8 per cent, respectively. The households had on an average 4.7 members. One-fifth of the selected households do not have any male member; 96 per cent of the surveyed households had one elderly person and around 3 per cent of households had two elderly persons. Around 90 per cent of the selected households had one widow, around 10 per cent of the households had two widows and only one household had three widows. More than half of the households were female headed.

Table 4.1

Selected Household Characteristics of the Surveyed Population

Selected Characteristics	*%*	*Number*
Household head		
Male	44.3	133
Female	55.7	167
Religion of household head		
Hindu	80.3	241
Muslim	7.0	21
Sarna*	12.7	38
Caste of household head		
Scheduled Castes (SCs)	14.3	43
Scheduled Tribes (STs)	40.0	120
Other Backward Classes (OBCs)	37.3	112
General Castes	8.3	25
Members in household		
Single member	13.7	40
2–4 members	36.7	110
5–8 members	43.7	131
More than 8 members	6.0	18
Number of aged persons in household (60+ years)		
One	96.0	288
Two	3.3	10
Three	0.7	2
Number of widows in household		
Single	90.0	270
Two	9.7	29
Three	0.3	1
Number of elderly widows in household		
One	99.3	298
Two	0.7	2
Total Number of Elderly Widows	**100.0**	**300**

* Details about *Sarna* Religion: Some western scholars and Indian sociologists refer to adivasi beliefs about the Sarna religion as *animism* and *spirit worship* and distinct from Hinduism, Christianity or Islam. In Jharkhand, Chhattisgarh and Odisha states, their religion is known as Sarna. As Orans (1965) reported, 'The movement is spoken of in the following terms': 'we should not leave our religion; we should continue to use rice-beer; we should have our worship at the sacred grove; also we should not stop eating beef. We will call our religion *Sarna Dhorom*' (pp: 113–119). The Jharkhand movement gave the Santhals (type of tribe) an opportunity to create a 'great tradition' of their own.

According to Troisi (2000), *Sarna* is the Munda word for 'sacred grove' while *Dhorom* is the Oriya word meaning 'religion'. Sarna involves belief in a great spirit called the *Sing Bonga*. Santhal belief holds the world to be inhabited by numerous spiritual beings of different kinds. Santhals consider themselves as living and doing everything in close association with these spirits. Rituals are performed under groves of Sal trees called *Jaher* (or *sacred grove*), where *Bonga* is believed to appear or express himself. Often *Jaher* are found in the forests.

Ownership of Agricultural Land

Table 4.2 presents the information on ownership of agricultural land for the surveyed households. Most of the households owned no land (55%). Further, a question was posed about the size of the land to those households who were having land. For the analysis purpose, based on the mean value of the land size, agricultural land and possession of irrigated land was classified as – marginal holders (land size less than and equal to 1.6 acre), small (1.61–2.4 acre) holdings, medium (2.41–3.2 acre) holdings and large (more than 3.21 acre) holdings. It was found that those who were having land, half of them were marginal holders. Little less than one-fourth (24.4%) of the households were having large holdings (land size more than 3.21 acre).

Majority of households were having irrigated land. Only 6 per cent were not having irrigated land. Further, to find out the income from the land, a question was asked – '*How much average yearly income are generated from your land?*' Twenty-three per cent of the households owning land reported no income from the land. Thirty-seven per cent of the households reported average yearly income from the land as more than ₹ 3500.

Table 4.2

Per cent Distribution of Surveyed Households by Ownership of Agricultural Land

Land Holdings	*%*	*Number*
Household owns any agricultural land		
Yes	45.0	135
No	55.0	165

Cont'd...

...Cont'd

Size of agricultural land		
Marginal (<= 1.6 acre) holdings	50.4	68
Small (1.61–2.4 acre) holdings	17.0	23
Medium (2.41–3.2 acre) holdings	5.9	8
Large (> 3.21 acre) holdings	24.4	33
Don't know	2.2	3
Possession of irrigated land		
Yes	91.9	124
No	5.9	8
Don't know	2.2	3
Size of irrigated land		
Marginal (<= 1.6 acre) holdings	48.9	66
Small (1.61–2.4 acre) holdings	15.6	21
Medium (2.41–3.2 acre) holdings	3.7	5
Large (> 3.21 acre) holdings	23.7	32
Don't know	2.2	3
Average yearly income from land		
No income	23.0	31
₹ 500–1,500	17.0	23
₹ 1,501–2,500	12.6	17
₹ 2,501–3,500	10.4	14
More than ₹ 3,500	**37.0**	**50**

Housing Characteristics

Table 4.3 provides information on ownership of house, housing quality, access to basic amenities, etc. In addition, information on main sources of lighting, cooking fuel, toilet facilities and drinking water were also collected. Majority of households (94%) owned the structure in which they resided. In case of the housing type, it was observed that about three-fifth of all households (59.7%) lived in *kachcha* houses (constructed from mud or other low quality materials), 16 per cent lived in semi-*pucca* houses and 24 per cent lived in *pucca* houses. More than half of the residential structures contained two to three rooms whereas 28 per cent of the residential structures consist of single room.

Only 40 per cent of the surveyed households had separate kitchen for cooking, around 30 per cent of the households cook inside their living rooms and 30 per cent of the households cook outside in open areas. Eighty-nine per cent of all surveyed households were using dry leaf/wood/coal/charcoal/dung cakes as main source of cooking fuel. Around 8 per cent of the households were using Liquid Petroleum Gas (LPG) and 3 per cent were using kerosene. Less than 1 per cent of the households were using electricity for the cooking purpose.

Seventy per cent of the surveyed households do not have access to the toilet facility. Less than one-third (28.3%) of the households were having pit toilet and 1 per cent of the households were sharing pit toilet. Majority of households (73%) had electricity for lighting. Around one-fourth of households were using kerosene as a main source of lighting. More than half of households (57%) reported that their main source of drinking water is public piped water/hand pump/covered well. Seventeen per cent of households use open well for drinking water. Only 16 per cent of households use own piped water, water from own hand pump or covered well.

Table 4.3

Per cent Distribution of Households by Selected Housing Characteristics

Housing Characteristics	*%*	*Number*
Own a house		
Yes	93.7	281
No	6.3	19
Type of house		
Kachcha	59.7	179
Semi-*pucca*	16.0	48
Pucca	24.3	17
Number of rooms in the house		
1	28.3	85
2–3	54.0	162
4–5	14.7	44
6 or more	3.0	9
Place for cooking food		
Inside living room	29.7	89
Separate kitchen	40.3	121
In an open area (outside the house)	30.0	40

Cont'd...

...Cont'd

Main type of fuel used for cooking		
Dry leaf/wood/crop residue/dung cakes/coal/charcoal	89.0	267
Kerosene	2.7	8
Electricity	0.7	2
LPG	7.7	23
Toilet facility in household		
Own flush toilet	0.7	2
Own pit toilet	28.3	85
Shared pit toilet	1.3	4
No facility	69.7	209
Main source of lighting in household		
Electricity	73.0	219
Kerosene	24.7	74
Oil*	2.3	7
Main source of drinking water in household		
Own piped water/hand pump/covered well	15.7	47
Own open well	10.0	30
Public piped water/hand pump/covered well	57.0	171
Public open well	17.3	52
Total Number of Elderly Widows	**100.0**	**300**

Note: * sesame oil or mustard oil

Households Benefitting from Government Schemes

It is evident from Table 4.4 that half of the surveyed households had below poverty line (BPL) cards and were receiving benefits. Among them, only six per cent of the households were not getting benefits of BPL card. Majority of the households were getting kerosene under the BPL card scheme followed by wheat (16.7%). Less than one per cent of the households were getting rice under BPL card. The reason given by Block Officer – '*they are not having enough rice or wheat to distribute among all the BPL households, so they distribute once in two to three months*'. It has been also found that 42 per cent of the households were having other cards. Among them, more than half (69%) of the households were having ration card and 15 per cent were having job card.

Table 4.4

Per cent Distribution of Households Benefitting from Government Schemes

Households Benefitting from Government Schemes	*%*	*Number*
Households having Below Poverty Line (BPL) card		
Yes	51.0	153
No	49.0	147
Households availing benefits under BPL card*		
Yes	94.1	144
No	5.9	9
Type of benefits		
Rice	0.7	1
Wheat	16.7	24
Sugar	1.4	2
Kerosene	81.3	117
Households with other cards		
Ration card (Antyodaya Card)	69.0	87
Voter identity card	9.5	12
Job card**	15.1	19
Green card (Above Poverty Line households)	6.3	8
Any family members receiving pension		
Yes	49.0	147
No	51.0	153
Type of pension being received		
Widow pension	74.1	109
Old age pension	19.0	28
Retired employee pension	5.4	8
Pension for disabled	1.4	2
Households benefitting from		
Indira Aawas Yojana	83.0	39
Toilet constructed out of government fund	14.9	8
Fund for house repair	2.1	1

Note: *Among those have BPL card.
** Card provided from the employment exchange.

Regarding pension, a question was posed to all households – *'Any member of the household receiving any type of pension?'* Among those who were getting pension, majority were receiving widow pension (74%) and 19 per cent were getting old age pension from the government. Five per cent of them were receiving pension for retired government employees and less than 1 per cent were receiving pension for disabled. To know whether the surveyed households were getting any other benefits from the government other than the pension, further probing was done – *'Any member of the family is getting any other benefits?'* Less than one-fifth (16%) of the households received other benefits such as Indira Aawas Yojana, followed by financial support to construct household toilets.

Remittances and Borrowing of Sampled Households

Another dimension of economic status of households is their borrowing/indebtedness. In order to examine this, a question was asked – *'Whether the household had borrowed money for any purpose during the last one year? If yes, what was the purpose of the money borrowed and the source of borrowing?'* Table 4.5 presents the remittances and borrowing of the sample households. Eight per cent of the surveyed households had members staying outside the village at the time of survey. Many among them were staying for employment purposes. More than half among them do not send any money to their houses.

Twenty-two per cent of the households had borrowed money during the last one year for various purposes. The most important reason mentioned was for health related expenses (37.9%), followed by meeting the household consumption (22.7%). Twelve per cent of the households borrowed money to meet marriage expenses of a family member. Major source of borrowing was neighbours (39.4%) and relatives (22.7%). Only 15 per cent have taken loans from banks and 14 per cent from local money lenders. Some respondents stated that if they borrow money from relatives or neighbours they need not pay any interest. Money lenders charge higher interest than banks. Thirty per cent of the households have indebtedness of around ₹ 700 to ₹ 2,000 whereas slightly less than one-fifth of the households have indebtedness of more than ₹ 8,500.

Table 4.5

Remittances and Borrowing of Sample Households

Sample Households	*%*	*Number*
Any member of household stays outside the village		
Yes	8.0	24
No	92.0	276
Purpose of staying outside the village*		
Study purpose	37.5	9
Job purpose	62.5	15
Does he/she sends money home*		
Yes	41.0	10
No	58.3	14
Dose this household borrowed money for any purpose		
Yes	22.0	66
No	78.0	234
Reasons for borrowing money**		
Health care/treatment	37.9	25
For marriage of son/daughter/sister/brother	12.1	8
For buying cow/tractor	3.0	2
For constructing/repairing house	6.1	4
For food/household consumption	22.7	15
For business/agriculture	18.2	12
Source of borrowing money**		
Money lenders	13.6	9
Bank	15.2	10
Relatives	22.7	15
Neighbours	39.4	26
Others (Employer/shopkeeper/friends)	9.1	6
Total indebtedness of the household**		
₹ 200 – ₹ 675	24.2	16
₹ 676 – ₹ 2,000	30.3	20
₹ 2,001 – ₹ 8,500	21.2	14
More than ₹ 8,500	24.2	16

Note: * Among those who stay outside the village.
** Among those who have borrowed money for any purpose.

Profiles of the Elderly Widows

Table 4.6 presents the distribution of respondents by selected socio-economic and demographic characteristics. In the present

Table 4.6

Distribution of Elderly Widows by Selected Socio-Economic and Demographic Characteristics

Background Characteristics	*%*	*Number*
Age group		
Young–old (60–69 years)	64.3	193
Old–old (70–79 years)	27.0	81
Oldest–old (80 and above years)	8.7	26
Religion		
Hindu	80.3	241
Muslim	7.0	21
Sarna*	12.7	38
Caste		
Scheduled Castes (SCs)	14.3	43
Scheduled Tribes (STs)	40.0	120
Other Backward Classes (OBCs)	37.3	112
Others	8.3	25
Literacy		
Literate	9.7	29
Non-literate	90.3	271
Number of sons		
No son	21.3	64
One son	28.3	85
Two sons	27.0	81
Three or more sons	23.3	70
Number of daughters		
No daughter	21.7	65
One daughter	26.7	80
Two daughters	24.0	72
Three or more daughters	27.6	83
Current work status		
Working	29.7	87
Not working	70.3	213
Occupational status**		
Non-agricultural labour	47.1	41
Agricultural labour	29.9	26
Self-employed/Petty business	20.7	18
Salaried	2.3	2
Total Number of Elderly Widows	**100.0**	**300**

Note: *Details given on pp. 56–57, ** For the working elderly widows only.

analysis, the age of elderly widows has been categorized as young-old, old-old and oldest-old, in the age groups of 60–69, 70–79 and 80 and above years respectively. Large proportion of the elderly widows is in the young-old age group (60–69 years) followed by old-old age group (70–79 years) and oldest-old age group (27% and 9%, respectively). Distribution by religion suggest that majority of the respondents were Hindus (80.3%), 13 per cent belong to the *Sarna* religion and 7 per cent were Muslims.

Forty per cent of the respondents were Scheduled Tribes (ST), followed by Other Backward Classes (37.3%). Scheduled castes (SC) and General Castes comprised 14 and 8 per cent respectively. Only 10 per cent of respondents were literate. Work status of the elderly widows indicates that around 30 per cent of them were engaged in one or other form of economic activity at the time of survey. Among them, 30 per cent of the elderly widows were engaged in agricultural work and 47 per cent were non-agricultural labourers, 21 per cent were self-employed and only 2 per cent were salaried employees.

Figure 4.1 shows the type of family of the respondents. More than half of the respondents (66.7%) were staying in nuclear families. One-fifth (20.3%) of the respondents were staying in joint families and 13 per cent were staying alone. Household's economic status, as measured by wealth index, composed of household asset data on ownership of selected durable goods. The wealth index has been constructed using principal component analysis (PCA). PCA is a multivariate statistical technique used to reduce the number of variables in a data set into a smaller number of dimensions (Vyas and Kumaranayake, 2006). As many as 15 items have been taken into consideration for the construction of wealth quintiles. The reliability co-efficient has been checked of these 15 items, which comes as 0.7954. Using the principal component analysis, factor score has been generated. The variables with positive factor scores are associated with high socio-economic status and variables with negative factor scores are associated with low socio-economic status. Subsequently, the households have been ranked and divided into quintiles – i.e., five groups, each containing an equal number of households. The first quintile represents households of the lowest (poorest) wealth status and the fifth quintile represents households with the highest (wealthiest) status and remaining are the middle groups.

The wealth quintiles suggests that slightly more than one-fourth (26%) of elderly widows belong to poorest households. About one-fifth (20%) were from richest households (Figure 4.1).

Figure 4.1

Per cent Distribution of Elderly Widows by Type of Family and Wealth Quintile

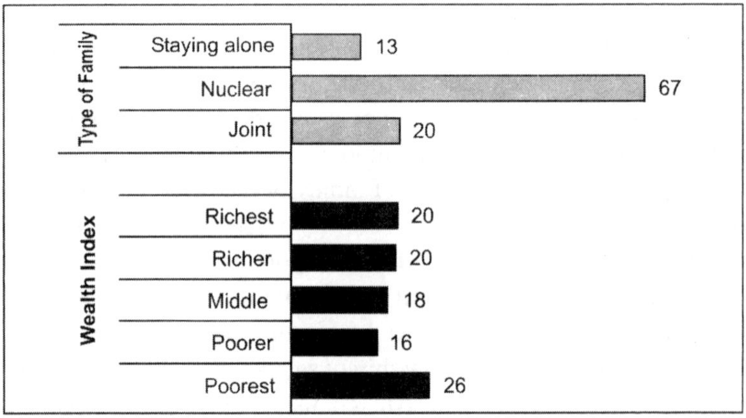

Further, a question was asked to the elderly widows – *'Was there any change in your place of residence after the death of your husband?'* Figure 4.2 shows three-fourth of respondents had changed their place of residence after widowhood. Those who have changed their place of residence after their husband's death, half of them were staying in nuclear families. However, 15 per cent of them were staying alone at the time of survey; 30 per cent were staying in joint families, who have changed their place of residence after widowhood.

Figure 4.2

Elderly Widows who have Changed their Place of Residence after Widowhood and Type of Family (%)

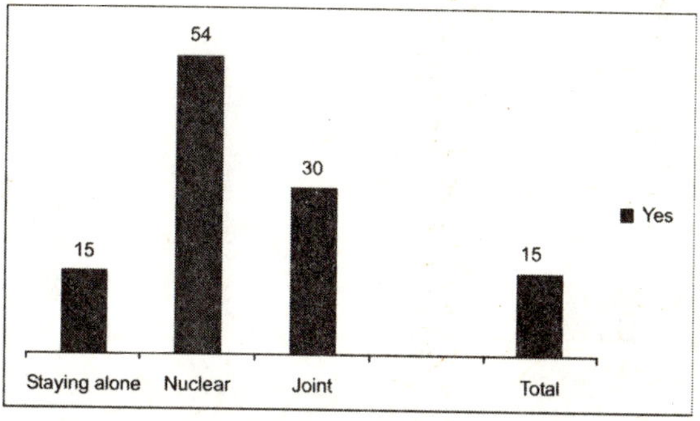

Age Gap between Husband and Wife

The particulars regarding the mean age at marriage of husband and wife and mean age gap between husband and wife are given in Figure 4.3. The mean age at marriage for husbands was 21.6 years and for wives, it was 12.9 years. The mean age difference between the spouses was 8.7 years.

Figure 4.3

Mean Age at Marriage of Husband and Wife and Age Gap between Husband and Wife (in years)

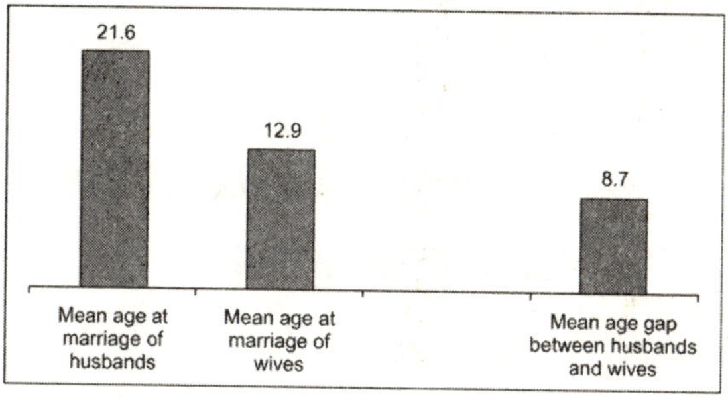

Age at Widowhood

The age at widowhood indicates that 7 per cent of the respondents have become widows when they were below 30 years of age, 38 per cent have became widows between the ages of 30 to 50 years. One-fifth of the elderly became widows after 60 years of age (Figure 4.4).

Figure 4.4

Age at Widowhood of Elderly Widows

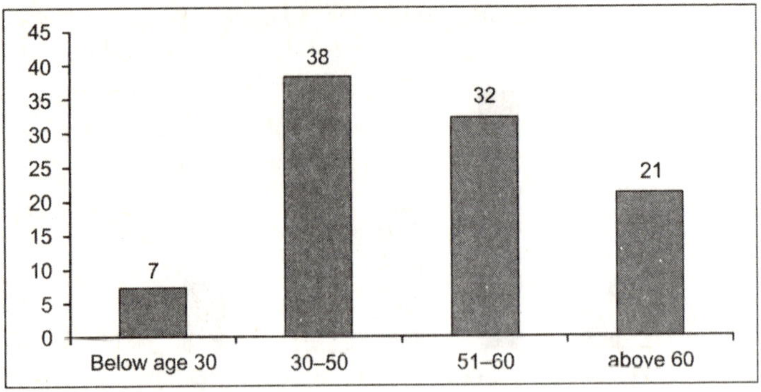

Duration of Widowhood

Mean duration of widowhood was 18 years. Nearly half (49.3%) of the respondents were widowed for a period of at least 11 to 20 years (Figure 4.5).

Figure 4.5

Duration of Widowhood and Mean Duration of Widowhood

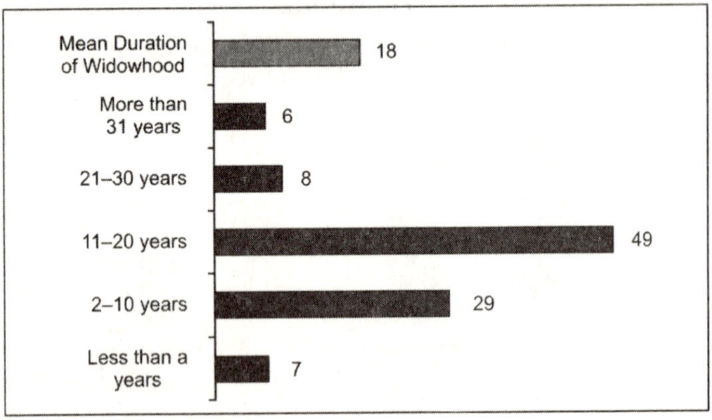

Note: Mean duration of widowhood (in years).

Rituals Performed for the Widows in the Study Villages

There are drastic changes in the lifestyle of women after widowhood. Widows have to start altogether a different life in dress, food habits, etc. Kitchlu (1993) found that there are some variations between different castes and religions. During the fieldwork, an attempt was made to understand the rituals performed during the widowhood in the study villages.

Rituals performed in the surveyed villages: In many traditional countries like India, widowhood represents a 'social death' for women. It is not only that they have lost their husbands, the main breadwinner and supporter of their children, but widowhood deprives them from their status and consigns them to the restrictions of society where they silently suffer the most extreme forms of discrimination and stigma.

Along with economic deprivation, when a woman becomes widow, stringent moral code is imposed on her, whereby her emotional and physical needs are not taken care of. When the husband is alive she is supposed to deck herself in colourful attire, wear ornaments and flowers, put *sindoor* and *kumkum*. But after the death of husband, she is doomed to live a life without any of these adornments. Widows are expected to remain in mourning during the remaining part of their life. She is expected to remain inside the home. She is forbidden to take part in any joyful occasion or to attend any family festival because her presence would be considered as inauspicious.

Rituals performed among some Hindus of surveyed villages: After the death of husband, all the family members assemble in the house. First they decorate the women whose husband has died and then they take the dead body for funeral. Relatives (widows) remove *sindoor* and break the bangles of the new widow. After that the widow takes bath in the river or pond and wears white saree and silver bangles. The white saree is a symbol of her widowhood. Three days after the death of husband, rice called 'Teeta Bhat', is prepared and distributed to all the relatives. Up to 10 days, the widow is not allowed to go outside the house.

Among backward castes of the study area, all rituals mentioned above are the same but there is one difference. After the funeral, the widow will be kept in a dark room for one night and nobody can see her face. In some communities after death of the husband, the widow needs to stay with another widow for 10 days. Some communities among Scheduled Castes of the study area, the new widow has to rub her forehead *sindoor* on the head of her dead husband. This shows that she has become a widow. After that, she is not allowed to wear any ornaments.

Among some Hindu communities, cooking is not allowed for three days after the death. Relatives or neighbours provide food for three days. On the eleventh day after death, all family members, including the widow, will take bath in the river. The widow will leave old cloths there and will wear a new dress, given from her parental house. Till eleventh day after the death, the house will be served food by another widow of the village and on the twelfth day, the family will give food, clothes and money to that widow. After the fourteenth day, the widow will go to her mother's house and will stay there for few days.

Rituals performed among the Muslims of surveyed villages: The nose pin worn during the marriage *(nikah)* is very important and will be removed after the death of the husband. Up to three days, perfumed oil will be applied in hair. On the third day, the widow will take bath and wear a white saree and bangle. On the tenth or fortieth day, family serves food to orphan children. Up to the fortieth day, widows are not allowed to go out.

About half of the elderly widows interviewed said that there are restrictions in the community for the widows. Some of the elderly widows stated that although there are no hard restrictions followed nowadays, but they themselves prefer to follow the old customs which they have seen for many years.

Summary

This chapter provides the characteristics of surveyed households and socio-demographic information of the elderly widows interviewed. Most of the surveyed households (80%) were Hindus, followed by 13 per cent belonging to the *Sarna* religion and 7 per cent were Muslims. Scheduled Tribes constitute 40 per cent of households. Around one-fifth of the surveyed households do not have any male member; 96 per cent of the surveyed households had one elderly person, around 3 per cent had two elderly persons and less than one per cent of households had three elderly persons. Ninety per cent of the selected households were having one widow and 10 per cent of the households were having two widows.

With regard to the household's ownership of the agricultural land it was found that most of the households (55%) owned no land. Less than one-fourth of households were having small land holdings (1.6 to 2.4 acre). Thirty-seven per cent of the households stated average yearly income from the irrigated land was more than ₹ 3500. Interestingly, 23 per cent of the households owning land reported no income from their land.

With regard to the housing characteristics of the surveyed households, majority of households (94%) owned the structure in which they resided. About three-fifth of the households (59.7%) lived in *kachcha* houses (constructed from mud or other low quality materials), 16 per cent lived in semi-*pucca* houses and remaining lived in *pucca* houses. Only 40 per cent of the households had a separate kitchen for cooking. Around 30 per cent of the households cook inside their living rooms The main source of cooking fuel was dry leaf/wood/coal/charcoal/dung cakes as reported by majority of the households. Around 8 per cent of the households were using Liquid Petroleum Gas (LPG) and 3 per cent were using kerosene. Seventy per cent of the households do not have access to a toilet facility. Slightly more than one-fourth (28.3%) of the households were having pit toilet facility.

Majority of households (73%) had electricity connection. Around one-fourth of households were using kerosene as main source of lighting. More than half of households (57%) reported that their main source of drinking water is public piped water/hand pump/covered well. Only 16 per cent of households use own piped water, water from own hand pump or covered well.

To understand whether the households were benefitted from any government programmes, the information was gathered about the type of government programmes/schemes availed by the households. Half of the surveyed households were having below poverty line (BPL) cards and were receiving foodgrains and kerosene meant for BPL card holders. Majority of the households were getting kerosene under the BPL scheme.

Among the surveyed elderly, around half of them were not receiving any pension. Those who were receiving pension, majority were receiving widow pension and 19 per cent were getting old age pension. The amount of widow as well as old age pension per month is ₹ 400. Five per cent among pensioners were receiving pension for retired employees. It was observed during the data collection that all the elderly widows were interested to avail pension from the government. When asked about the reasons for not getting the pension, they stated that many do not know how to apply, or officers told them to wait, or they are not eligible for the pension.

To understand the household's economic condition, questions were asked to the heads of the households that whether they have borrowed money from any source. Finding suggests that 22 per cent of the households had borrowed money during the last one year. The most important reason mentioned was treating health problems, followed by meeting the household consumption. Twelve per cent of households had borrowed money to meet marriage related expenses. Neighbours are the major source for borrowing money, followed by relatives. About 15 per cent took loans from banks and 14 per cent depended on local money lenders, who charges higher interest.

About 64 per cent of the elderly widows were in the young-old age group (60–69 years); 27 per cent of them were in the old-old age group and 8 per cent were in oldest-old age group. Religious composition suggests that majority of the respondents were Hindus, while 40 per cent of the respondents belonged to the Scheduled Tribes. Majority of the elderly widows were non-literates. Work status of the elderly widows indicates that around 30 per cent of them were engaged in one or other form of economic activity at the time of survey. Among them, 30 per cent of the elderly widows were engaged in agricultural work and 21 per cent were self-employed. Many elderly widows were working as maids in households.

More than half of the respondents (66.7%) were staying in nuclear families. It is important to mention here that 13 per cent of elderly widows were staying alone. Household wealth index suggests that slightly more than one-fourth (26%) of elderly widows belong to the poorest households. Three-fourth of the respondents revealed that they have changed their place of residence after widowhood. Half of those who were staying in nuclear families at the time of data collection had changed their place of residence after husband's death. Seven per cent of the respondents have become widow before 30 years of age whereas one-fifth of them became widow after 60 years of age. Nearly half of the respondents were widowed for a duration of at least 11 to 20 years.

5

Living Arrangements and Economic Status of Elderly Widows

In India, family is the primary care-giver for elderly persons and acts as a principal source of support and security in old age. Living arrangements of the elderly, where the older people live and with whom they live, make a significant difference to a variety of factors that may directly or indirectly contribute to the quality of their life (Prakash, 1999). India is still characterized by its traditional ways of living where several generations of a family live together within the same household. Traditional living arrangements wherein elderly live with their children and extended families. These arrangements are a form of social safety net for them in the absence of social security schemes or private pension plans (Choudhuri and Roy, 2009).

Due to the effect of modernization, westernization and urbanization in our society, the traditional bonds with the extended family members are now gradually breaking. The elderly have been the biggest sufferers of the changing values in the family system in India. The living arrangements of the elderly have been severely affected by disturbing the multigenerational familial co-residence and compelling them to live by themselves as elderly couple or alone, if widowed (Audinarayana and Kavitha, 1997). Widowhood is the event which constitutes the greatest change in the family status of older people (Arling, 1976). Living arrangements are influenced by a variety of factors, including marital status, financial well-being, health status and family size and structure, as well as cultural traditions such as kinship patterns, the value placed on living independently or with family members, the availability of social services and social support (Velkof, 2001).

In the Indian context, it is not only the number of children available but their gender and marital status that also determines the co-residence pattern. Audinarayana and Kavitha (1997) found that number of surviving sons exhibit a positive association with the living arrangements of widows. Elderly widows have to suffer from many problems. Of all problems, the financial one is the most crucial. The economic status of the elderly is determined by four factors – their employment status, their access to state pensions, their access to private savings and their receipt of financial support (Stark, 1954).

One of difficulties faced by the widows is economic subsistence and the management of resources. Sometimes widows tend to adjust their economic situation by seeking employment, even if they are very old and not healthy. The absence of savings and social security compels most of the widows to continue to work as long as they can. The widows who have no savings or pension benefits have to depend on their sons, daughters or other relatives for their livelihood. Given this background, this chapter analyses the living arrangements, economic conditions, level of economic dependency, pension benefits, ownership of land and house, etc. of the elderly widows.

Living Arrangements of Elderly Widows

Living arrangements become an important constituent of the overall well-being and also provides some indications of the level of actual support available to the elderly (Rajan and Kumar, 2003). The distribution of elderly widows by their actual living arrangements is presented in Table 5.1. With regard to living arrangements of elderly widows, nearly 15 per cent of the elderly widows were living with their unmarried children. More than half of the respondents were living with their married sons compared to only 6 per cent living with married daughters. This clearly reflects the typical characteristics of a patrilineal society, i.e. the cultural norm of elderly parents living with sons. The cultural practice of daughters going to their husbands house after marriage, while sons remain as members of their parental households even after marriage, is still a dominant practice in rural India.

Table 5.1

Per cent Distribution of Elderly Widows according to Current Living Arrangements

Living Arrangements	*Percentage*	*Number*
Living alone	13.0	39
Living with unmarried children	14.7	44
Living with married son	55.3	166
Living with married daughter	6.0	18
Living with other relatives	11.0	33
Number of Elderly Widows	**100.0**	**300**

The elderly widows live with married sons either together in a large household or adjacent to it. When this preferred arrangement is not possible, then the elderly widows prefer to co-live with others. It was found that 11 per cent of elderly widows were living with their relatives i.e. with brother, sister, grandchildren, etc. Table 5.1 also highlights that 13 per cent of the elderly widows are staying independently without any direct support from family members. On the other hand, living alone does not mean that potential support is altogether non-existent to the elderly widows. But, it indicates that the amount of support is likely to be lower and the degree of loneliness and social isolation is also likely to be higher as compared to those who are living with children or other relatives (Panda, 1997). It is also an indication that the traditional family system is gradually changing in India, even in remote rural areas.

Table 5.2 presents the background characteristics of elderly widows by their current living arrangements. Age of the elderly is one of the major determinants of living arrangements. More than half (52.8%) of the young-old (60–69 years) widows were staying with their married sons compared to only 6 per cent of elderly widows of same age group staying with their married daughters. Around 12 per cent of young-old widows were living alone.

Among the old-old category (70–79 years), majority were living with their married sons. Among the oldest-old (80+ years) widows, 15 per cent were living alone and around four per cent were living with other relatives. The living arrangements of the elderly widows by caste group reveals that while more than one-fifth (23.3%) of the elderly widows belonging to the Scheduled Castes were living alone, only 8 per cent of the elderly

Table 5.2

Per cent Distribution of Elderly Widows by Actual Living Arrangements according to Selected Background Characteristics

Background Characteristics	*Living Alone*	*With Unmarried Children*	*With Married Son*	*With Married Daughter*	*With Other Relatives*
Age group					
Young–old (60–69 years)	11.9	19.2	52.8	5.7	10.4
Old–old (70–79 years)	14.8	7.4	55.6	7.4	14.8
Oldest–old (80+ years)	15.4	3.8	73.1	3.8	3.8
Religion					
Hindu	14.1	11.2	57.3	6.6	10.8
Non-Hindu	8.5	28.8	47.5	3.4	11.9
Caste					
SCs	23.3	7.0	51.2	9.3	9.3
STs	15.8	19.2	47.5	6.7	10.8
OBCs	7.1	13.4	66.1	2.7	10.7
Others	8.0	12.0	52.0	12.0	16.0
Number of Sons					
No son	29.7	14.1	NA	18.8	37.5
One son	4.7	7.1	78.8	4.7	4.7
Two sons	13.6	21.0	61.7	0.0	3.7
Three and more sons	7.1	17.1	70.0	2.9	2.9
Number of Daughters					
No daughter	26.2	6.2	40.0	NA	27.7
One daughter	8.8	15.0	58.8	13.8	3.8
Two daughters	8.3	18.1	59.7	4.2	9.7
Three and more daughters	10.8	18.1	60.2	4.8	6.0
Total	**13.0**	**14.7**	**55.3**	**6.0**	**11.0**

Note: NA indicates not applicable.

widows belonging to the general castes were living alone. It is generally believed that in traditional societies like India, children are considered as security during old age. Irrespective of the age, living with married son is the most common living arrangement observed. Elderly widows who were not having a son, majority of them either lived alone (29.7%) or living with other relatives (37.5%). As expected, the number of sons was negatively associated with the elderly living alone.

In India, son is considered as the most important care provider for elderly parents. It is evident from the bi-variate analysis that the number of sons is negatively associated with elderly widows living alone. For example, only 5 per cent of the elderly widows lived alone when they had one son whereas 30 per cent of the elderly widows lived alone when they did not have a son. The proportion of elderly widows living alone has declined with an increase in the number of sons. Similarly, the proportion of elderly widows living with other members also declined with an increase in the number of sons they have.

The number of daughters is also equally important in determining the living arrangements for elderly widows. It can be seen from Table 5.2 that 26 per cent of the elderly widows living alone when they did not have a daughter. This is one of the indications of the importance of sons in determining the living arrangements of the elderly widows. Other studies also supported the view that the number of children positively related to the probability of living with them (Bian, 1998; Burch and Mathews, 1987; Martin, 1989; Rajan and Kumar, 2003; Zimmer and Kwong, 2003).

Table 5.3 shows who is the decision-maker about the current place of residence for the elderly widows. The data reveals that among those who are currently living alone, 23 per cent of elderly widows said that their children took the decision in this regard. However, for majority, it was their own decision to stay alone. Those who are currently living with their married children or grandchildren, among them 33 per cent said that their children took the decision and in 9 per cent of cases, the decision was made by their relatives.

Table 5.3

Per cent Distribution of Elderly Widows by Living Arrangements and Persons took the Decision

Decision by	*Actual Living Arrangements*			
	Living Alone	*With Unmarried Children*	*With Married Children or Grandchildren*	*With Other Relatives*
Self	69.2	81.8	58.1	14.3
Children	23.1	18.2	33.0	7.1
Other relatives	7.7	0.0	8.9	78.6
Number of Elderly Widows	**39**	**44**	**203**	**14**

Table 5.4

Elderly Widow's Perception about Current Living Conditions and Actual Living Arrangements (% distribution)

Perception on Current Living Conditions	*Actual Living Arrangements*			
	Living Alone	*With Unmarried Children*	*With Married Children or Grandchildren*	*With Other Relatives*
Comfortable	46.2	63.6	52.2	50.0
Satisfactory	17.9	18.2	35.0	42.9
Uncomfortable	35.9	18.2	12.8	7.1
Number of Elderly Widows	**39**	**44**	**203**	**14**

A question was asked to the elderly widows – '*How do you feel about your current living condition?*' The responses were broadly categorized into three – *comfortable, satisfactory and uncomfortable*. Table 5.4 shows that those who were living alone, among them 46 per cent felt that their current living condition is comfortable. Around 36 per cent said that their current living condition is uncomfortable. More than half (63.6%) of the respondents who were living with their unmarried children were comfortable, 18 per cent of them said that they were satisfied. However, equal per cent of elderly widows were uncomfortable with their current living conditions. Of the elderly widows who are living with their married children or grandchildren, more than half were comfortable with their current living condition. Only 13 per cent of elderly widows expressed being 'uncomfortable' to stay with their married children or grandchildren.

While interviewing, an elderly widow said – '*After the death of my husband I suffered a lot. After two years of my son's marriage, my daughter-in-law started quarrelling with me. She never gives me enough food*'. Further she mentioned – '*For whom I was doing all the hard work all these years, now treats me like this! My son and daughter-in-law will throw me out one day*'.

Table 5.5

Per cent Distribution of Elderly Widows according to Opinion on Current Living Conditions by Selected Background Characteristics

Background Characteristics	*Opinion on Current Living Conditions*		
	Comfortable	*Satisfactory*	*Uncomfortable*
Age group			
Young–old (60–69 years)	53.9	31.6	14.5
Old–old (70–79 years)	51.9	28.4	19.8
Oldest–old (80+ years)	50.0	30.8	19.2
Number of sons			
No son	48.4	32.8	18.8
One son	52.9	31.8	15.3
Two sons	55.6	27.2	17.3
Three and more sons	54.3	31.4	14.3
Number of daughters			
No daughter	46.2	33.8	20.0
One daughter	55.0	28.8	16.3
Two daughters	52.8	30.6	16.7
Three and more daughters	56.6	30.1	13.3
Occupational status *			
Non-agricultural labourer	46.3	29.3	24.4
Agricultural labourer	74.1	14.8	11.1
Self-employed/Petty business	47.4	21.1	31.6
Salaried	100.0	0.0	0.0
Type of family			
Single	46.2	17.9	35.9
Nuclear	51.5	33.5	15.0
Joint	62.3	29.5	8.2
Number of Elderly Widows	**159**	**92**	**49**

Note: * This information pertains to only those who are presently engaged in any economic activity (N = 87).

The Table 5.5 shows the background characteristics of the elderly widows by their opinion about the current living conditions. More than half of young-old widows reported as comfortable with their current living conditions. However, 15 per cent were uncomfortable. Among the old-old categoıy, slightly more than one-fourth (28.4%) were satisfied and around one-fifth (19.8%) were uncomfortable with their current living conditions. Among the oldest-old widows, 31 per cent expressed satisfaction with the current living conditions.

Among the elderly widows who were not having a son, 48 per cent were comfortable, 33 per cent were satisfied and 19 per cent were uncomfortable with their current living conditions. Having a son in a way ensures support during old age. Among the elderly widows having one son, more than half of them were comfortable with their current living condition. As the number of sons increases the proportion who report as 'comfortable' also increases. It was observed that of the elderly widows having three or more daughters, more than half were comfortable with their current living conditions.

According to the occupational status of elderly widows, 11 per cent of the elderly widows who were agricultural labourers reported as 'uncomfortable' with their current living conditions. Those who were self-employed, more than one-fourth (31.6%) stated that their current living condition is uncomfortable. Elderly widows working as non-agricultural workers, 29 per cent were satisfied and 24 per cent were uncomfortable with their current living conditions.

Family is the most important social unit and also the major source of care and support to the aged, especially for widows. About one-third of elderly widows living alone mentioned their living conditions as 'uncomfortable', and one-fifth (17.9%) expressed satisfaction on the current living conditions. Those who were staying in nuclear families, nearly half of them were comfortable with their present living conditions. Of the elderly widows from joint families, majority were satisfied with their current living conditions.

Table 5.6

Per cent Distribution of Elderly Widows according to Preferred Living Arrangements and Actual Living Arrangements

Arrangements	*Preferred Living Arrangements*				
	Living Alone	*With Unmarried Children*	*With Married Sons*	*With Married Daughters*	*With Other Relatives*
Living alone	66.7	0.0	23.1	2.6	7.7
Living with unmarried children	9.1	81.8	9.1	0.0	0.0
Living with married son/s	7.8	0.6	91.0	0.6	0.0
Living with married daughter/s	0.0	0.0	5.6	94.4	0.0
Living with other relatives	15.2	0.0	9.1	0.0	75.8

A question was posed to elderly widows about their preference in living arrangements. Among the elderly widows who were currently living alone, 67 per cent prefer to live alone and little less than one-fourth (23.1%) want to live with their married sons. Among the respondents who are currently residing with their married sons, majority prefers to live with them. However, 8 per cent prefer to live alone. Of the elderly widows who were currently living with their married daughters, only 6 per cent prefer to live with their married sons. Among those who were currently living with other relatives, 15 per cent prefer to live alone (Table 5.6).

To understand the factors that influence preference for living arrangements, the actual living arrangement and the stated preferences were compared. Around 47 per cent of the respondents stated that there was nobody to take care of them. Thirty-five per cent of elderly widows said that it is very difficult to manage everything at this stage of their life. Five per cent stated that their daughters-in-law were not supporting them (Figure 5.1). As one old lady narrated her problem – '*My daughter-in-law always tries to find fault with me. Even if my son is eager to keep me with him, she is not allowing. What can I do*?' Around 13 per centalso stated other reasons such as, 'they don't have son/daughter', 'it is not good to stay with a married daughter', etc.

Figure 5.1

Reasons for the Difference between Actual Living Arrangements and Preferred Living Arrangements

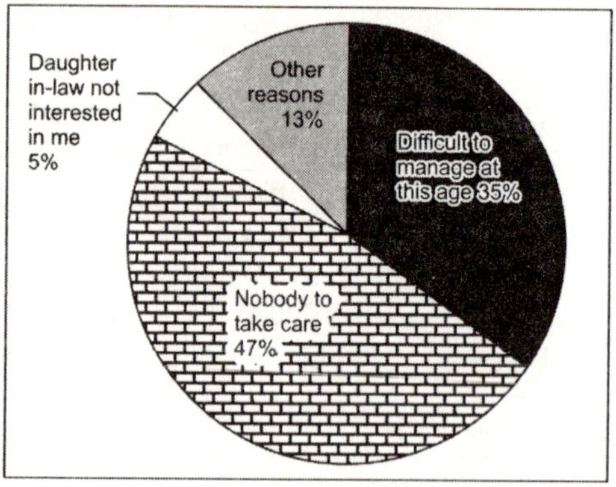

Widowhood is a stage in life when a woman faces several difficulties after the death of her husband. Family members do not want to keep her. Sometimes, they blame the widow for the death of the man. Because of several problems, a widow is forced to leave the house. In this context, it is important to know whether the widows had changed their place of residence after the death of their husbands. About 15 per cent of the elderly widows had changed their place of residence after the death of their husbands. About 13 per cent of elderly widows from nuclear families have changed their residence. Slightly less than one-fifth (23%) of elderly widows who were currently staying in joint families had changed their place of residence after their husband's death (Table 5.7).

Table 5.7

Respondents who have changed their Place of Residence after Husband's Death by Type of Family (%)

Type of Family	*Change in Place of Residence after Husband's Death*	
	Yes	*Number of Elderly Widows*
Living Alone	17.9	39
Nuclear Family	12.5	200
Joint Family	23.0	61
Total	**15.3**	**300**

The reasons given by the elderly widows for the change in the place of residence shows that majority of them (44%) felt that, after the death of their husbands, nobody wanted to keep them. Thirty per cent said that they were alone, so they have to move to other place. Around 9 per cent of the elderly widows who have changed their place of residence after their husband's death said that their sons started working in other places, so they also moved with them.

Figure 5.2

Reasons for Change in Place of Residence after Husband's Death

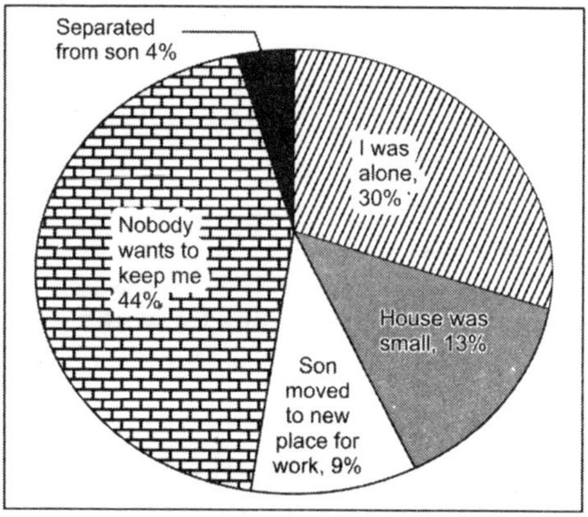

Economic Status of Elderly Widows

The elderly expect economic, social and emotional support from family members. Their economic productivity and physical strength decline considerably with advancing age. Economic factors are major determinants of well-being. The economic position of widows has been an important concern in many societies. In societies in which the husband was typically the sole provider, his sudden death could plunge his family into poverty and crisis. After the death of husbands, many widows were forced to take up work. This was entirely a new experience for many women since they always lived under the protective cover of their partner. Economic necessities compel many elderly to continue to work with lower wages and in an unhealthy and hazardous environment, to take care of themselves and to support those directly depending on them (Sekher, 2005). Table 5.8 shows that more than half (66%) of the elderly widows were engaged in some income earning activity. However, only one-fourth (29%) of them were working at the time of survey.

Table 5.8

Per cent Distribution of Elderly Widows according to Work Status and Type of Work

Work Status	*%*	*Number*
Ever worked		
Yes	66.0	198
No	34.0	102
Currently working		
Yes	29.0	87
No	71.0	213
Type of work*		
Non-agricultural labourer	47.1	41
Agricultural labourer	29.9	26
Self-employed/Petty business	20.7	18
Salaried	2.3	2
Whether receiving cash as remuneration for work*		
Yes	88.5	77
No	11.5	10

Note: *Among those who are currently working (N = 87)

Though majority of these elderly widows who work outside earn some money, few receive grains (rice) as remuneration. In few cases, it was observed that women work outside only to get food. Since most of these women work in agriculture and informal sector, the wages are very low. The average wage of a women agricultural worker is ₹ 30, whereas the male worker gets about ₹ 50 per day. The availability of these jobs is seasonal.

Majority of young-old (60–69 years) widows were currently working. As age increases, the proportion of working elderly widows decreases, which is evident from Table 5.9. However, 15 per cent of elderly widows in the age group of 70–79 years were still working. More than half (54%) of the elderly widows among Scheduled Tribes were working. However, only 7 per cent of the elderly widows from general category were working at the time of the survey. Majority of elderly widows who were currently working were non-literates. Elderly widows having no son or daughter were more among the workers. According to the type of family, 68 per cent of elderly widows who were currently working were from nuclear families. Twenty four per cent elderly widows who live alone reported as working.

Table 5.9

Elderly Widows Engaged in an Economic Activity according to Selected Background Characteristics (%)

Background Characteristics	*Percentage*
Age group	
Young-old (60–69 years)	85.1
Old-old (70–79 years)	14.9
Oldest-old (80+ years)	0.0
Religion	
Hindu	81.6
Muslim	4.6
Sarna*	13.8
Caste	
SC	18.4
ST	54.0
OBC	20.7
General	6.9
Literacy status	
Literate	3.4
Non-literate	96.6
Number of son/s	
No son	31.0
One son	25.3
Two sons	32.2
More than two sons	11.5
Number of daughter/s	
No daughter	32.2
One daughter	26.4
Two daughters	20.7
More than two daughters	20.6
Type of family	
Single	24.1
Nuclear	67.8
Joint	8.0
Number of Elderly Widows	**87**

Note: * Sarna is a religion meaning animism and spirit worship and is distinct from Hinduism, Christianity or Islam (details are given in Chapter 4 pp. 56–57).

Figure 5.3

Reasons for Taking-Up the Work (%)

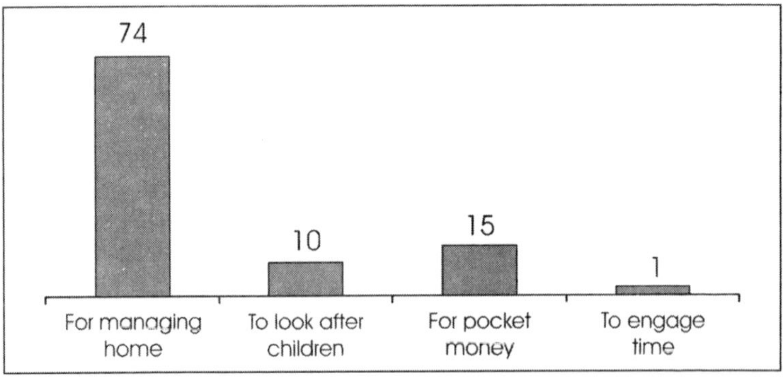

Further, elderly widows were asked – '*Why are you still working outside your home, even at this advanced age?*' Nearly three-fourth of them was forced to work to manage the household requirements. One-tenth among elderly widows continues to work to support their children. Fifteen per cent of elderly widows were working to earn '*pocket money*', which they can spend for themselves. Only 1 per cent of elderly widows stated that they are working to engage time (Figure 5.3). After husband's death, elderly widows had to take the responsibility of earning and managing their households as well as maintaining children. Whatever little amount of money they earned was needed to support the family.

More than half (51.7%) of elderly widows were getting ₹ 101 to ₹ 500 in a month for their work, about one-fifth (19.5%) were getting ₹ 501 to ₹ 1,000 and around 13 per cent were getting ₹ 30 to ₹ 100 in a month for their work. Only 5 per cent of elderly widows were getting more than ₹ 1,000 in a month for their work. In an interview with the Sarpanch of one study village (key informant interview – Annexure B), he said:

> People prefer to keep old widows in their houses because they are ready to work even for no wages (just for food). Another reason for keeping elderly widows as maids is they are available full time in the house. Young maids prefer to take up work in many households to earn more.

Dependency Level of Elderly Widows

Widowhood brings dependency, especially at the later age, when she does not have any economic assets or regular income. In that case, widows have to fully depend on others for their day-to-day survival. In order to probe these aspects, a question was asked to the elderly widows – *'Are you economically dependent on others?'* The responses were grouped into three broad categories – *fully dependent on others, partially dependent, and not dependent*. Table 5.10 illustrates that around two-fifth (40.3%) of elderly widows are fully dependent on others for economic support. Around 18 per cent are partially dependent and 42 per cent are not dependent on others.

Table 5.10

Per cent Distribution of Elderly Widows by Level of Economic Dependency

Economic Dependency Level	*%*	*Number*
Fully dependent	40.3	121
Partially dependent	17.7	53
Not dependent	42.0	126
Number of Elderly Widows	**100.0**	**300**

Figure 5.4

Source of Income for Economically Independent Elderly Widows (%)

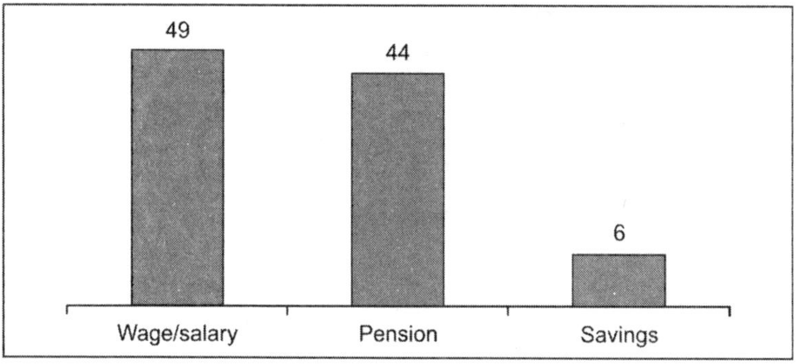

Further a question was asked to those who are not economically dependent on others: How do they meet their economic needs?' About half of them were working to meet their day-to-day needs, 44 per cent were meeting their needs through pension and 6 per cent were using their savings for their requirements (Figure 5.4).

Table 5.11

Level of Economic Dependency according to Actual Living Arrangements of Elderly Widows (%)

Actual Living Arrangements	Level of Economic Dependency		
	Fully Dependent	Partially Dependent	Not Dependent
Living alone	5.1	0.0	94.9
Living with unmarried children	50.0	18.2	31.8
Living with married son	44.0	21.7	34.3
Living with married daughter	61.1	11.1	27.8
Living with others	39.4	21.2	39.4

In this study, an attempt was made to understand the dependency levels of elderly widows according to their living arrangements. It is evident from Table 5.11 that out of the elderly widows who are living alone, majority are not dependent on others for economic support. However, 5 per cent are still dependent on others for their day-to-day maintenance. Elderly widows who are living with their unmarried children, nearly half of them are fully dependent and 18 per cent are partially dependent for financial requirements. Those who are living with their married sons, 34 per cent are not economically dependent. However, around 44 per cent are fully dependent on others. Elderly widows who are living with their daughters also show higher levels of economic dependency.

Economic Support to Elderly Widows

Family is the prime care-giver for overwhelming proportion of aged in India. Multigenerational living arrangements have been an integral part of the rural social life. However, due to migration of youngsters, changing attitudes and lifestyles, several young adults prefer to live in nuclear families even in rural areas. This shift in the attitude leaves many older women to fend for themselves, particularly after the death of their husbands.

Sometimes family members economically support the elderly widows and sometimes they do not. Elderly are no longer considered as productive and useful. For many, an elderly widow is a burden on the family. So, it is important to know who is supporting the widows for their economic requirements. Table 5.12 presents the persons financially supporting the elderly widows. Majority (45%) of the economically dependent elderly widows were supported by their sons. Thirty per cent of elderly widows stated that they are managing on their own. Interestingly, 12 per cent of elderly widows were depending on their daughters for financial support. Few receive financial support from their siblings.

Table 5.12

Persons Supporting Economically Dependent Elderly Widows

Persons Financially Supporting	*%*	*Number Elderly Widows*
Self	30.0	90
Depending on son	45.0	135
Depending on daughter	12.3	37
Depending on son-in-law	3.7	11
Depending on siblings	2.3	7
Depending on others	6.9	20
Total	**100.0**	**300**

However, around 36 per cent were not satisfied with the economic support that they are receiving presently from family members.

What are the reasons for not being satisfied with the family members for their economic support? Forty three per cent of the elderly widows, who were not satisfied with the economic support from their family, said that the money does not fulfil all their needs. Thirty seven per cent stated that family does not give anything to them. Seven per cent of elderly widows felt that family members do not really care for them. Nine per cent of elderly widows revealed that their sons have their own family to support, whereas four per cent said that their sons are not working and not in a position to support (Figure 5.5).

Figure 5.5

Reasons for not being Satisfied with the Economic Support from Family

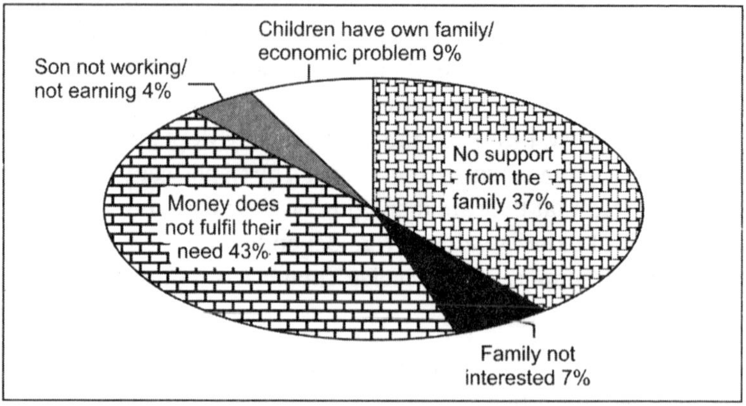

As one elderly widow said – *'Nowadays, everyone wants to stay in a small family of husband and wife. Nobody wants their old parents to stay with them. Especially if one becomes widow, then nobody is there to take care of her'*. Further she said – *'Duniya janti hai ki pati rahne se sabhi puchhte hai, baad mein koi nahi puchhta hai'*, (Everyone knows in this world, if husband is alive then everyone will ask about you, otherwise nobody even thinks of you).

Access to Money

To understand the access to financial resources among elderly widows, information was obtained on whether they had any savings, owned an account in a bank or post office and if so, whether they operated their own accounts. The findings are presented in Table 5.13.

More than half (53.7%) of the elderly widows have an account in a bank or post office. With regard to the operation of the account, around 79 per cent of widows operated it themselves. Seventeen per cent needed the help of either children or grandchildren to operate the account. Although more than half of the elderly widows were having an account in a bank or post office, but majority do not have any savings.

Table 5.13

Percentage of Elderly Widows having an Account in a Bank/Post-office, Operating the Account and having any Savings

Account in a Bank/Post Office	*%*	*Number*
Yes	53.7	161
No	46.3	139
Who operates your account *		
Self	78.9	127
Children/Grand Children	16.7	27
Others**	4.4	7
Any savings in Bank/Post office*		
Yes	16.8	27
No	83.2	134
Total	**100.0**	**161**

Note: *Among those who have an account either in a bank or in post office
**Others include son-in-law, brothers/sisters, village head, etc.

India does not have a universal social security system to protect the elderly against economic deprivation. Half of the surveyed elderly widows were not receiving any pension. Those who were receiving pension, majority (72.8%) were getting widow pension and around one-fifth were getting old age pension. About seven per cent were getting employee pension (for retired persons) and only 1 per cent were getting pension for the disabled.

Block Development Offer stated the reasons for not getting pension as – '*There are many elderly and widows who have applied for pension, but when pension department enquires, most do not have proper documents. Many of them even do not have their age proof certificate*'.

The state and central governments have a provision to distribute pension every month. Elderly widows were asked – '*Whether they receive pension regularly?*' Majority (65.3%) received their pension once in every four months. Only 8 per cent stated that they are receiving pension every month.

More than half of the elderly widows who are getting pension go alone to receive the pension, 38 per cent take somebody with them to go to pension office and around 9 per cent receives pension through *'gram sevak'* or village officials. More than half of those who were receiving pension stated that the pension money does not fulfil their requirements and is not sufficient. About 45 per cent of elderly widows use their pension for their own personal needs.

Table 5.14

Elderly Widows Receiving Pension

Receiving pension	*%*	*Number*
Yes	49.3	147
No	50.7	153
Type of pension*		
Old age Pension	19.0	28
Widow Pension	72.8	107
Employee Pension	6.8	10
Other (Disabled)	1.4	2
Frequency of receiving the pension*		
Every month	8.2	12
Once in every two months	11.6	17
Once in every four months	65.3	96
Once in every six months	15.0	22
How you collect the pension*		
Go alone	53.1	78
Take somebody's help	38.1	56
Through gram sevak/village officials	8.9	13
Whether pension money fulfil your requirements*		
Yes	42.9	63
No	57.1	84
What you do with the pension money*		
Using for food for self	4.8	7
Using on medicines for self	6.8	10
Buying cloths for self	0.7	1
Giving to house	42.9	63
Using for own needs	44.9	66

Note: *Among those who receive pension (N= 147).

The amount of old age pension and widow pension is only ₹ 200 per month. The Block Development Officer of surveyed area revealed that earlier pension was distributed in cash but now they have opened a bank account for all pensioners and directly money goes to their account. He further said – *'Because of this, aged or widows need not to give any money/bribe to middle men'*.

Ownership of Land and Property

According to the existing practice in the study area, land was usually inherited from father to son. According to customs, a widow possessed rights over the land of her deceased husband until her sons were mature enough to manage the family property.

Table 5.15

Ownership of House and Land by Elderly Widows

Any house in the name of elderly widow	%	*Number*
Yes	18.0	54
No	82.0	246
Ownership of the house		
Self	18.0	54
Father-in-law	15.0	45
Husband	39.0	117
Son	16.0	48
Brother-in-law	3.3	10
Others	8.6	26
Does your household have any land?		
Yes	49.0	147
No	51.0	153
Ownership of land*		
Self	24.5	36
Father-in-law	12.9	19
Husband	34.0	50
Son	22.4	33
Brother-in-law	2.0	3
Others	4.1	6

Note: *Among those who own land (N= 147)

Table 5.15 presents ownership of land among elderly widows. Eighty-two per cent of elderly widows do not have a house in their name and half of the elderly widows do not own any land. When the question was asked about the ownership of the house in which she was currently living, 39 per cent of the elderly widows said that the house is in the name of her deceased husband. Only 18 per cent of elderly widows had ownership of the house in which she was residing. Fifteen per cent of elderly widows said that her father-in-law was the owner of the house. A sizeable proportion of elderly widows stated that their sons are the real owners of the house.

Table 5.16

Inheritance of Land and House by Elderly Widows

*Inheritance of land from parents***	*%*	*Number*
Yes	9.5	14
No	90.5	133
Inheritance of land from husband**		
Yes	50.3	74
No	49.7	73
Persons taking care of land		
Self	16.3	24
Son/Daughter-in-law	46.3	68
Daughter/son-in-law	3.4	5
Brother-in-law	12.9	19
Relatives	11.6	17
Others	9.5	14
Inheritance of house from parents		
Yes	2.0	3
No	98.0	144
Inheritance of house from husband		
Yes	23.8	35
No	76.2	112

Note: ** Among those who own any land (N =147)

Table 5.16 illustrates that among the elderly widows who own land, only nine per cent inherited land from their parents and half of them inherited from their husbands. When it comes to taking care of the land, very few (16%) elderly widows were managing their land. Sons are the major care-takers of land. Around 13 per cent of elderly widows said that their brothers-in-law are taking care of the land. One in 10 elderly widows said that they have given their land to others for managing. Regarding the inheritance of house, only 2 per cent of elderly widows inherited house from their parents. Slightly less than one-fourth of widows (23.8%) inherited land from their husbands.

Summary

This chapter provides information on living arrangements and economic status of elderly widows. Majority of elderly widows had no income and were economically dependent on others. Living arrangements indicates that a large proportion of elderly widows are living with their married sons.

According to Indian social system, sons are expected to take care of parents in their old age. But the traditional family structure is slowly breaking down since last few decades even in rural areas. This has led to a situation in which many elderly are forced to mend themselves and live alone. According to the study, 13 per cent of the elderly widows were living alone. This is an indication of their changed status in the family after becoming widow.

As children are considered to be an old age security, parents depend on their children for economic, physical and emotional support. Analysis shows that 23 per cent of elderly widows reported that their children took decision regarding their present living arrangements.

As it is important to know the living arrangements of the elderly widows, it is also important to know their satisfaction about the current living conditions. Elderly widows living with their married children (son/daughter) or grandchildren were comfortable with present living conditions compared to those who were living alone. Number of children also determines the living arrangements of elderly widows. As the number of son or daughter increases, more elderly widows reported their living condition as comfortable. This may be because they are getting support, care, love and respect from sons or daughters and this fulfils most of their needs. It was also found that some of the elderly widows were not so happy with their present living arrangements but they were forced to stay. More than two-fifth of elderly widows have changed their place of residence after their husband's death, as nobody from their family wanted to keep them.

Most of the elderly widows were economically dependent on others. Those who were not economically dependent on others, most of them earn some money to fulfil their needs. Among the elderly widows who were economically not dependent, 44 per cent were using pension to meet their necessities. Less than one-tenth of elderly widows were using their savings for their requirements.

It is also important to know the persons supporting the elderly widows. Majority (45%) of economically dependent elderly widows was depending on their sons and most of them were satisfied with the extent of economic support received from their sons.

Access to money is one of the important dimensions to assess the status of elderly widows. It was found that more than half of elderly widows have an account in a bank or in a post office and around four out of five operate it themselves. The bank account is mainly used for receiving the pension. Majority of elderly widows do not have any savings. Most of the respondents were getting widow pension with a monthly payment of ₹ 200. Regarding the ownership of land and house, survey revealed that 82 per cent of elderly widows do not have a house in their name and half of elderly widows do not have any land in their names. The inheritance of the property shows that elderly widows who own land, only 9 per cent were inherited from their parents and half of them inherited the land from their husbands. Sons are the major care-takers of the land.

6

Health Status and Treatment Seeking Behaviour of Elderly Widows

Health status is an important factor that has bearing on almost every single aspect of our lives, particularly for the aged. World Health Organization has defined health as a 'state of complete physical, mental, and social well-being and not merely the absence of disease or infirmity'. It can determine what activities or tasks one can or cannot engage in. Health can also influence the way we perceive ourselves. Apart from the economic problems, there are non-economic problems associated with the widowhood. A study in Bangalore (Prakash, 1998) found that the fear of physical dependency, including being sick or disabled, was the major cause of worry for the elderly. We have limited understanding of the relationships, both direct and indirect, between health and living arrangements. Several studies have found that older adults living together with family members have better subjective well-being than those living alone (Chen and Silverstein 2000; Chen and Short 2008; Wu and Schimmele 2008).

When thinking about the health of the elderly, it is important to consider not only the objective measures of health such as the incidence of chronic disease or functional disability, but also psychological health and well-being. The available information on physical and psychological health status of elderly widows of the study area was examined here. To measure the physical health status of the elderly widows, the health outcomes such as self-reported health status were considered. Self-reported health status describes how a person perceives his or her own health and is also an indicator for the well-being or quality of life. Quality of life undergoes changes over lifespan and health becomes one of the major concerns, especially in old age. Measure of functioning ability assessed by activities of daily living provides a social definition of health in terms of departure from normal role function (Waweru et al., 2003).

Scales have been developed to measure the physical and psychological health of the elderly widows. To measure the overall health status of the elderly widows, 'health adjustment inventory' was used. For measuring the psychological health condition of the elderly widows, 'Geriatric Depression Scale (GDS)' was employed in this study.

Health Conditions of Elderly Widows

The general characteristics of the old age are the physical and psychological changes and very often it is associated with disability. It is often seen that aging is accompanied by multiple illnesses and physical ailments. The health status occupies the central place in any study of elder population.

The elderly face number of health problems and adjust to those conditions in varying degrees in their old age. These problems become manifold when it is related to the widows in the absence of social security, loss of social role and recognition, and also non-availability of care-givers. Widowhood is also associated with poverty for many, which increases the health risks.

Perception about Health Conditions

General health conditions of the elderly widows were examined here. Figure 6.1 shows that 41 per cent of the elderly widows felt that their health condition is fair. However, 28 per cent of elderly widows reported that they were having poor health. However, one-fifth (20%) of the elderly widows consider their health condition is very good or good. Around 11 per cent of the elderly widows believe that their health condition is very poor.

Figure 6.1

Percentage of Elderly Widows according to Perceived Health Conditions

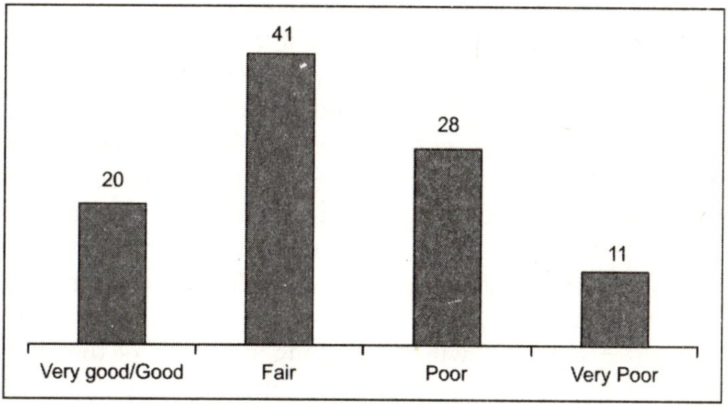

Table 6.1

Per cent Distribution of Elderly Widows by Perceived Health Conditions according to Background Characteristics

Background Characteristics	*Very Good*	*Fair*	*Poor*	*Very Poor*	*X^2 Values*
Age group					
Young-old (60–69 years)	21.8	40.9	31.1	6.2	
Old-old (70–79 years)	18.5	44.4	22.2	14.8	18.4
Oldest-old (80+ years)	11.5	34.6	23.1	30.8	
Number of sons					
No son	18.8	50.0	23.4	7.8	
One son	25.9	32.9	35.3	5.9	13.5
Two sons	19.8	44.4	23.5	12.3	
Three and more sons	14.3	40.0	28.6	17.1	
Work status					
Currently working	21.8	51.7	20.7	5.7	9.0
Currently not working	19.2	37.1	31.0	12.7	
Type of family					
Single	28.3	46.2	12.8	12.8	
Nuclear family	18.5	39.5	33.0	9.0	10.0
Joint family	19.7	44.3	21.3	14.8	
Dependency level					
Full dependent	19.0	34.7	33.1	13.2	
Partially dependent	15.1	60.4	22.6	1.9	14.0
Not dependent	23.0	39.7	25.4	11.9	
Total	**20.0**	**41.3**	**28.0**	**10.7**	

According to the findings presented in Table 6.1, around 41 per cent of young-old widows reported their health condition as fair compared to only 6 per cent who reported it as poor. Slightly less than one-fifth (18.5%) of old-old widows perceived their health condition as very good or good as compared to 15 per cent of those who reported their health conditions as very poor. Forty-four per cent of old-old widows felt that their health condition is fair. Less than one-fifth (15%) of old-old widows had very poor health conditions, as compared to 18 per cent who reported very good or good health condition. Among the oldest-old widows, about 31 per cent felt that their health condition is very poor.

In the category of windows having sons, half of the elderly widows having no son reported their health condition as fair, only 8 per cent of them reported poor health condition. Work status of elderly widows revealed that those who were working at the time of survey, slightly more than half (51.7%) of them have reported fair health condition. Slightly more than one-fifth (21.8%) of working elderly widows had either very good or good health condition as compared to one-fifth who perceived their health condition as poor. Among the elderly widows who were not working at the time of survey, around 13 per cent had reported very poor health conditions.

Around 47 per cent of elderly widows staying alone felt their health as fair and more than one-fourth (28%) stated their health as very good or good. Health status of elderly widows from nuclear families shows that around 19 per cent felt their health as very good or good, 33 per cent perceived it as poor and 9 per cent consider it as very poor. Majority (40%) of elderly widows perceived their health condition as fair. Fifteen per cent felt their health was very poor. Slightly more than one-fifth (21.3%) felt that their health condition is poor. Those who are not economically dependent on others, among them around 40 per cent have fair health condition.

Analysis revealed that elderly widows who perceive their physical health as very good or good, majority among them were comfortable with their current living conditions. Around three-fourth of elderly widows who perceive their physical health condition as very poor were also uncomfortable with their current living conditions (Table 6.2).

Table 6.2

Elderly Widows according to Perceived Health Status and Current Living Conditions (%)

Perceived Health Status	*Current living Conditions*			*Number of Elderly Widows*
	Comfortable	*Satisfactory*	*Uncomfortable*	
Very good/good	61.7	31.7	6.7	60
Fair	53.2	25.0	21.8	124
Poor	50.0	34.5	15.5	84
Very poor	43.8	40.6	15.6	32
Total	**53.0**	**30.7**	**16.3**	**300**

Disability among Elderly Widows

Census 2001 data shows that two out of every five disabled aged 60 years and above are widowed. According to Rajan et al. (2005), widows constitute a vulnerable group and widowhood consist a much greater risk factor for the aged women as compared to men. Priya (2007) by analysing 58th Round of NSSO data concluded that access to resources is less for widowed women compared to men. Present study examines the types of disabilities among the elderly widows of the study area. It also examined the dependency, employment status, general education level, living arrangements of disabled elderly widows. Table 6.3 shows that 43 per cent of the elderly widows were having disability at the time of the survey. Among the disabled elderly widows, more than half (68%) suffer from at least one form of disability and 32 per cent were having more than one disability.

Among the disabilities reported, the proportion of elderly widows who were having problem in vision is the highest (55%), followed by problem in walking (35%). Nine per cent of the disabled elderly widows reported problem in hearing. Only 13 per cent of the disabled elderly widows use physical impairment aid. Most of them use aid for improving vision and stick for walking. Only five per cent of disabled elderly widows use aid for hearing impairments.

Table 6.3

Per cent Distribution of Elderly Widows by Type of Disability

Disability	*Percentage*	*Number*
Elderly widows with physical impairments		
Yes	43.3	130
No	56.7	170
Number of disability*		
One	67.7	88
More than one	32.3	42
*Elderly widows having difficulty in**		
Hearing	9.2	12
Visual	55.4	72
Walking	35.4	46
Using aid for the disability*	13.0	39
Elderly widows who use aid for		
Hearing	5.1	2
Vision	69.2	27
Walking	25.6	10

Note: *Among those who reported any disability (N= 130).

What are the reasons for not using aid for their disabilities? Forty-one per cent of elderly widows have reported that they do not have money for buying the aid, whereas one-fourth of them said that aid will not be useful to overcome the disability (Figure 6.2). Slightly more than one-fifth (22%) reported that there is no

Figure 6.2

Reasons for not using Aid for Impairment (%)

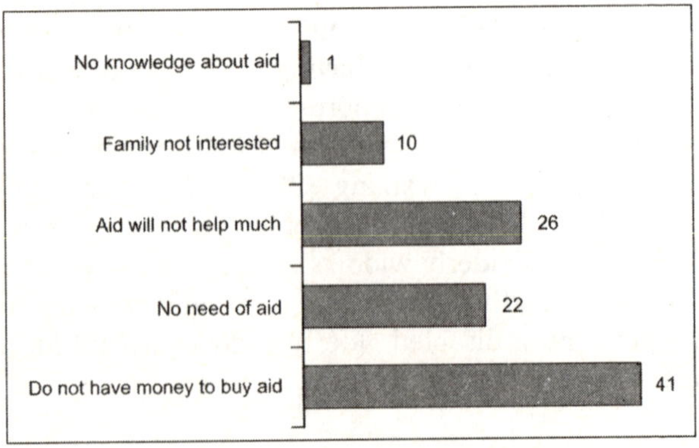

need of any aid for their disability that is why they are not using it. One out of ten elderly widows stated that their family is not interested in providing the aid. Few elderly widows said that they do not have any knowledge about the aid that can be used for minimizing the disability and from where to get it.

Majority of the elderly widows (57%) stated that their sons are meeting the expenses to purchase the aid for their disability. Ten per cent of disabled elderly widows get money from their daughters for buying aid and 33 per cent are managing themselves (Figure 6.3).

Figure 6.3

Persons Meeting the Cost of Aid for Impairment

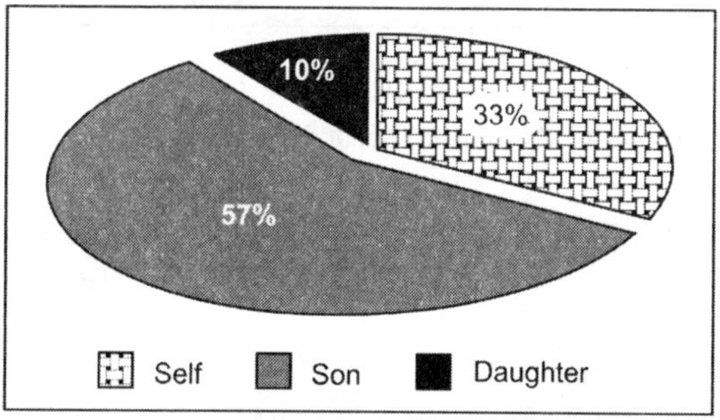

Disability and health status of elderly widows were analysed to understand the reported health status of the disabled elderly widows. Table 6.4 shows that among those who had hearing problems, half of them had reported their health as poor. Forty-three per cent of elderly widows with vision problems felt that their health was fair, 33 per cent felt it as poor and 15 per cent reported their health as very poor. Majority of elderly widows with difficulty in walking reported their health status as poor.

Advancing age is associated with the increasing prevalence of diseases and disability. Among the three age categories (young-old, old-old and oldest-old) of elderly widows, the problem of vision was more reported as compared to other two problems i.e. hearing and walking (Figure 6.4). Among the young-old widows, one in 10 had hearing problem, around 41 per cent had difficulty in walking and 49 per cent had difficulty in vision. Among the old-old widows, more than half had visual problems. Among the oldest-old widows, 55 per cent had vision problems followed by difficulty in walking.

Table 6.4

Per cent Distribution of Elderly Widows according to Types of Disability and Perceived Health Status

Perceived Health Status	*Type of Disability*		
	Hearing	*Visual*	*Walking*
Very good/Good	16.7	8.3	2.2
Fair	16.7	43.1	28.3
Poor	50.0	33.3	41.3
Very Poor	16.7	15.3	28.3
Total	**9.2**	**55.4**	**35.4**

Figure 6.4

Elderly Widows by Age Group according to Types of Disability (%)

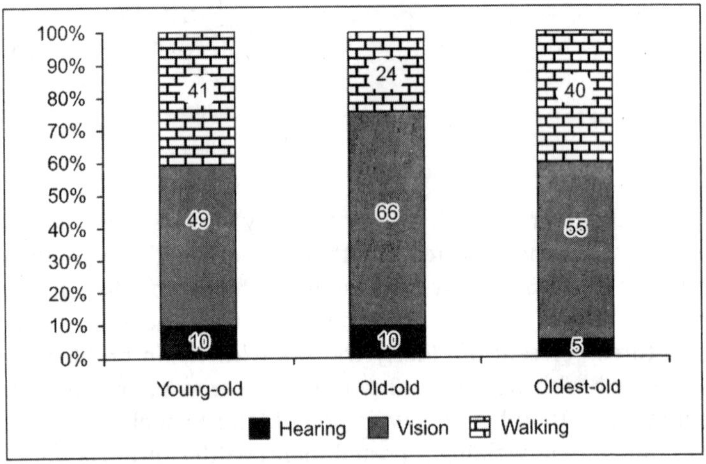

Health Problems among Elderly Widows

An attempt has been made to understand the prevailing diseases among the elderly widows of the study area. A question was asked to all elderly widows – *'Are you suffering from any sickness/health problem?'* If the response was *yes,* further it was asked, *'What type of sickness you have?'* Finding suggests that three-fifth of elderly widows were suffering from health problems at the time of the survey.

General weakness, blood pressure, joint pain and gastrointestinal problems were reported by large proportion of elderly widows. Sizeable number of elderly widows also reported other health problems which include anaemia, paralysis, ulcer, tumour, and asthma.

Table 6.5

Percentage Distribution of Elderly Widows by Types of Disease

Disease	*Percentage*	*Number*
Blood pressure	15.5	28
Heart problems	1.7	3
Tuberculosis	1.7	3
Gastrointestinal	16.6	30
Joints pain	21.5	39
General weakness	33.1	60
Other diseases*	10.0	18

Note: Among those who reported diseases (N= 181).

**Other diseases includes: Anemia, Paralysis, Ulcer, Tumour, Asthma, Filaria,*

Figure 6.5

Elderly Widows with Self-Reported Health Problems (%)

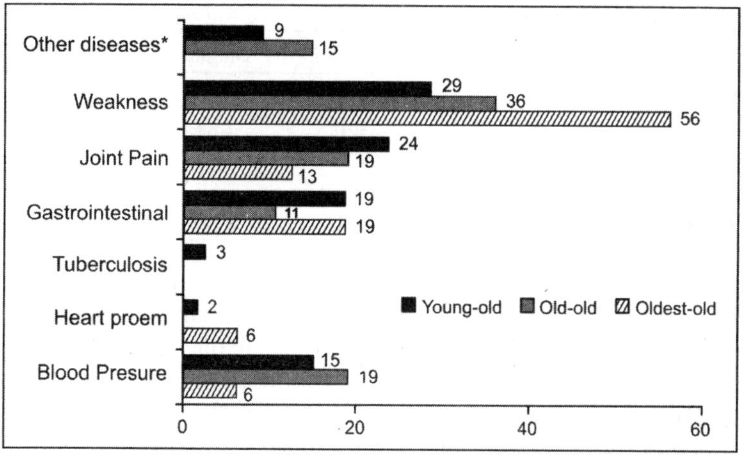

Note: Among those who reported as having diseases (N= 181).

* Other diseases include: anaemia, paralysis, ulcer, tumour, asthma, filariasis.

Figure 6.5 presents the prevalence of selected health problems as reported by elderly widows. Disease pattern according to the age of elderly widows shows that most of the oldest-old widows reported weakness as a major health problem. Blood pressure among the old-old widows is high compared to other two categories. Other diseases (*anaemia, paralysis, ulcer, tumour, asthma,* and *filariasis*) among the old-old widows are high than in the young-old widows.

Co-morbidity or the combination of multiple health problems is a challenging situation for the elderly. The study examines the risk of having multiple health problems among the elderly widows. Table 6.6 summarizes the combined prevalence of reported health problems by the elderly widows according to their age groups. Around 31 per cent of elderly widows in the oldest-old category reported as having three or more health problems compared to 16 per cent among young-old widows. Interestingly, about 39 per cent of oldest-old widows did not report any health problems.

Table 6.6

Percentage of Elderly Widows with Multiple Health Problems

Number of Health Problems	*Age-Group*		
	Young-old	*Old-old*	*Oldest-old*
No health problem	38.9	42.0	38.5
One	24.4	28.4	11.5
Two	21.2	14.8	19.2
Three and more	15.5	14.8	30.7
Percentage Elderly Widows	**64.3**	**27.0**	**8.7**

Sometime it happens that certain diseases are more severe but may not create immediate difficulty. For example; if a person is having both blood pressure and joint pain, although blood pressure is more dangerous but it may not be creating problem always. On the other hand, joint pain will cause immediate problem. In that case, joint pain is perceived by the patient as more severe than the blood pressure. It all depends on the person that how s/he experiences and perceives the problem. To examine this, the surveyed elderly widows who reported as having two or more health problems were asked to rank their health problems according to the severity. Table 6.7 presents the diseases as reported by the elderly widows. Blood pressure is ranked one by around 30 per cent of elderly widows having two or more diseases, followed by joint pain (27%) and general weakness (18%). Asthma and diabetes were also ranked as one by around 4 and 3 per cent of elderly widows, respectively. On the other hand, elderly widows having two or more health problems, joint pain is ranked as second most severe problem by 35 per cent of elderly widows. Around 30 per cent ranked blood pressure in second order, followed by general weakness (19%).

Table 6.7

Percentage of Elderly Widows Reporting the Most Severe Disease

Disease Ranked 1	*Percentage*	*Disease Ranked 2*	*Percentage*
Blood pressure	29.6	Blood pressure	26.9
Diabetes	2.8	Diabetes	0.9
Joint pain	26.9	Joint pain	35.2
General weakness	17.6	General weakness	19.4
Heart problems	2.8	Heart problems	0.0
Asthma	3.7	Asthma	2.8
Gastrointestinal	12.0	Gastrointestinal	8.3
Others*	4.6	Others*	6.5

* Other diseases include: anaemia, paralysis, ulcer, tumour, filaria.

Duration of the prevalence of disease were also collected from the elderly widows which shows that the occurrence of most severe disease among most of them were about three to six years. Less than one-fifth of elderly widows were suffering during the last one year or one to three years.

Table 6.8

Percentage of Elderly Widows according to Duration of Disease

Disease 1	*Percentage*	*Disease 2*	*Percentage*
Last one year	16.7	Last one year	13.9
One to three years	18.5	One to three years	27.8
Three to six years	35.2	Three to six years	39.8
Seven years and more	29.6	Seven years and more	18.5

Physical Mobility and Functional Disability

The health related quality of life of the elderly, especially for women, is considerably lower in India when compared to other countries (Gupta et al., 2001). Information on physical mobility of the elderly widows was collected. Physical mobility is an important indicator of physical condition of health and is also an indication of the degree of dependence on others for movement and performing daily routine. The physical mobility of the elderly widows was categorized into three – *physically immobile, confined to bed, and confined to home*. It was found that majority of the elderly widows (69.3%) were physically mobile. However, 30 per cent were confined to home and less than one per cent were confined to bed (Table not shown). To study the well-being of elderly, one of the approaches is to study their *'competence'* in daily living. Such competence assesses the ability to manage the tasks of daily living without depending on others. Disability is a complex phenomenon that manifest in many ways and evolves over a longer time span. It refers to an individual's inability to perform basic household activities such as eating, dressing, cooking, bathing, walking, etc. Under this situation, an individual can be described as 'disabled' if her/his personal capabilities fall less than is actually demanded by his/her own environment or family conditions (Alam and Mukherjee, 2003).

Functional disability was measured in terms of self-reported disability in routine daily activities which is understood by answering the following questions – *'Do you require any help or support for: getting out of bed, bathing, walking for some distance, taking food, dressing, going to toilet, and cooking?'* The answers were coded into three categories – *no need of any help, need help and can't do even with help.*

Table 6.9 presents the activities of daily living (ADL) among the elderly widows. It shows that around one-fifth of elderly widows need help for walking, 17 per cent require help for going to toilet, 14 per cent were dependent on others for getting out of bed and 16 per cent can't cook food for self even with the help. This shows the extent of physical dependency of elderly widows for understanding their day-to-day activities.

Table 6.9

Percentage of Elderly Widows by Activities of Daily Living (ADL)

Daily Activities (ADL)	*No Need of Any Help*	*Need Help*	*Can't do Even with Help*
Getting out of bed	86.3	13.7	0.0
Bathing	90.7	9.3	0.0
Walking for some distance	74.0	26.0	0.0
Eating	97.3	2.7	0.0
Dressing	94.7	5.3	0.0
Toileting	83.3	16.7	0.0
Cooking	71.7	12.3	16.0

Treatment Seeking Behaviour of Elderly Widows

Seeking treatment for health problems is also a matter of accessibility and affordability. The elderly widows of the study area were asked about their treatment for the diseases. Analysis revealed that three-fourth of the elderly widows sought treatment for their health problems. However, one-fourth among them was not seeking medical treatment for various reasons.

Figure 6.6

Elderly Widows Taking Treatment for Health Problems

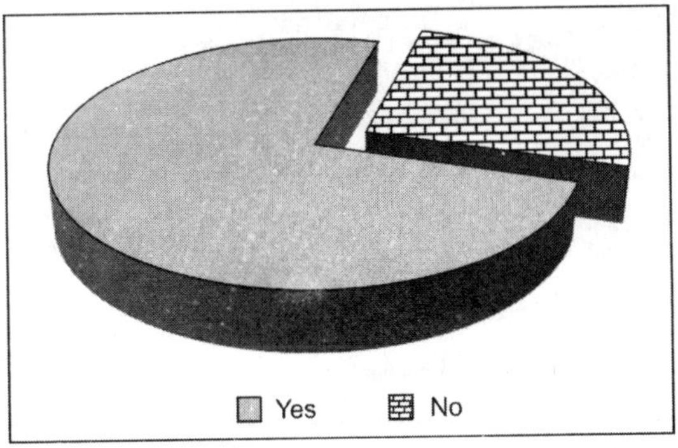

The reasons given by the elderly widows for not seeking treatment for their health problems have been given in Figure 6.7. Many elderly widows revealed that they do not have the money for the treatment. Thirty-seven per cent perceive that treatment will not work at this age, and around seven per cent said that their children are not really interested in arranging their treatment.

Figure 6.7

Reasons for Not Seeking Treatment for Health Problems

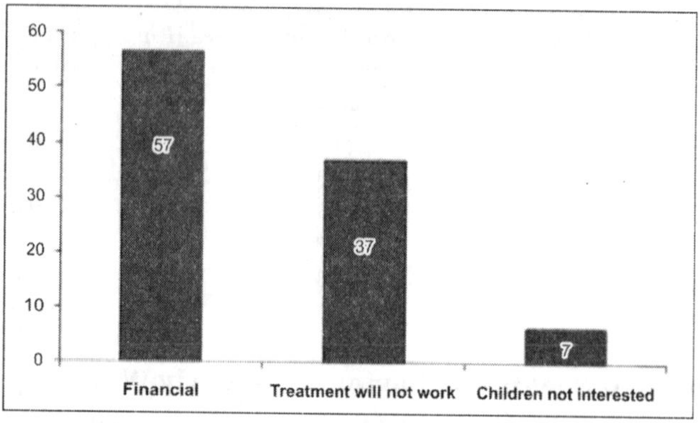

Further, it was asked about the place of treatment. More than half of them were taking treatment from private hospitals, followed by 31 per cent from government hospitals. Five per cent of elderly widows were depending on traditional healers (Figure 6.8).

Figure 6.8

Place of Treatment for Health Problems

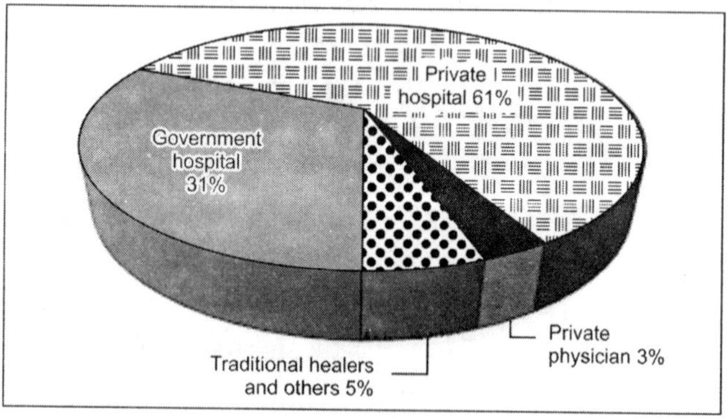

The social system in India puts pressure on individuals to look after the old, particularly the elderly widows. A question was asked about the care-taker of the elderly widows when they are sick. Nearly half of the respondents were taken care of by their sons and daughters-in-law. One-fifth were taken care of by their daughters during ill health.

According to this study, on an average ₹ 333 was spent for the treatment by the elderly widows in a month. Information about the persons meeting the cost of the treatment was also collected. It was found that around half of the elderly widows were supported by their sons or daughters-in-law for health treatment whenever needed. Thirty-nine per cent of elderly widows were managing themselves to meet the treatment cost. Less than 10 per cent of elderly widows were getting support from their daughters or sons-in-law for meeting the medical expenditure.

Table 6.10

Money Spent for Treatment and Persons Meeting the Cost of Treatment

Money Spent for Treatment	*Percentage*	*Number*
Monthly expenditure on treatment		
Less than ₹ 150	32.6	45
₹ 150 to ₹ 300	37.7	52
More than ₹ 300	29.7	41
Average monthly expenditure on treatment	₹ 333.11	
Persons meeting the cost of treatment when required?*		
Self	38.5	52
Son/Daughter-in-law	49.6	67
Daughter/Son-in-law	8.2	11
Brother/Others**	3.7	5

Note: *Among those who are getting treatment (N=135).
** Others include: grandchildren, sister, brother-in-law, etc.

Table 6.11

Elderly Widows according to Economic Status of Households and Place of Treatment (%)

Economic Status of Households	*Place of Treatment*				*Number of Elderly Widows*
	Government Hospital	*Private Hospital*	*Chemist/ Drug Store*	*Traditional Healers/ Others*	
Poorest	48.0	48.0	0.0	4.0	25
Poorer	50.0	38.9	5.6	5.6	18
Middle	28.0	56.0	4.0	12.0	25
Richer	22.2	72.2	0.0	5.6	36
Richest	19.4	74.2	6.5	0.0	31
Total	**31.1**	**60.7**	**3.0**	**5.2**	**135**

Further, economic status of households and place of treatment were analysed. Majority of elderly widows belonging to the poorest households were taking the treatment from government hospitals. Three-fourth of the elderly widows belonging to richer households went to private hospitals. Only 19 per cent took treatment from government hospitals.

Health Adjustment Inventory for Elderly Widows

To measure the overall health status of elderly widows, the 'Health Adjustment Inventory for the Elderly' was utilized. The adjustment inventory was constructed by Bell (1934) and further it was standardized for Indian situation by Ramamurthy (1968). The inventory measures the interaction of the elderly with the environment (i.e. home, family and other social activities and interaction outside home). The inventory has 66 items and is grouped into different sub-scales – family adjustment, social adjustment, emotional adjustment, self-adjustment and health adjustment. The sub-scale health adjustment inventory has 14 items. To understand the overall situation of health, a composite health index including 14 items were computed. Some questions were positive and some were negative in nature. After checking the reliability with alpha values (0.8427), the composite index has been computed by giving a value of one for positive indicator and zero for otherwise. In case of negative statements, value one has been given for negative response and zero for otherwise. The total score ranging from 0 to 14 indicates the degree of adjustment in health dimension. High score indicates poor health adjustment and low score indicates good health adjustment. On the basis of total scores and the mean value of the score, the index has been categorized into three – *'good' (0–5 score), 'moderate' (6–10 score), and 'poor' health adjustment (11 and above).*

Health Adjustment among Elderly Widows

The distribution elderly widow on health adjustment inventory is presented in Figure 6.9. This shows that 45 per cent of the elderly widows are having 'moderate' health adjustment, followed by around 38 per cent were having 'good' health adjustment. According to this inventory, 17 per cent of elderly widows were having 'poor' health adjustment.

Figure 6.9

Health-Adjustment Inventory for Elderly Widows

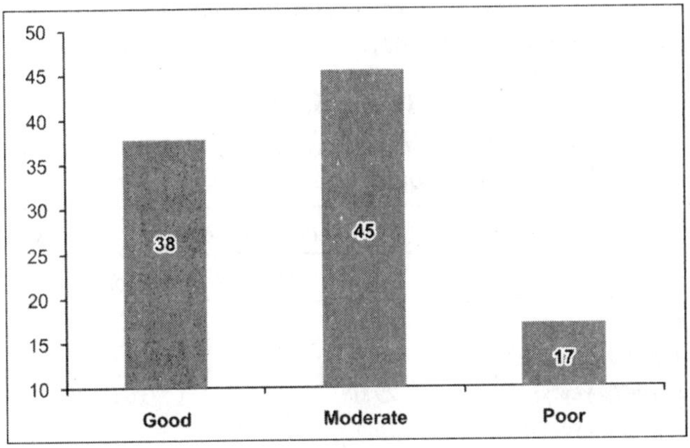

Elderly widows' health adjustment also depends upon their age, number of children, type of family, economic dependency and health status. Here, an attempt has been made to understand the health adjustment among the elderly widows according to certain characteristics. Chi-square test was done to find out the association between the background variables and the health adjustment. Table 6.12 explains the health adjustment inventory among elderly widows according to background characteristics.

Age and current health status were emerged as significant factors at 1 per cent level of significance. Current work status and economic dependency was significant at 5 per cent level of significance. It indicates that with increasing age, elderly widows have significantly poor adjustment with health. Young-old widows' health adjustment is good as compared to that of old-old and oldest-old widows.

The findings revealed that number of sons do not have any significant impact on the health adjustment of elderly widows. This may be because sons are busy with their family and other works and they are not getting time to take care of the health of their elderly mothers.

Work status and health adjustment were found to be in a significant relationship with each other. Majority among working elderly widows have moderate level of health adjustment. According to the type of family, among those who were living alone, slightly less than one-fourth were reported poor health adjustment compared to those who were from joint families. No significant association was observed between the type of family and health adjustment of elderly widows.

Table 6.12

Health-Adjustment Inventory among Elderly Widows according to Background Characteristics

Background Characteristics	*Health-Adjustment*			*X^2 Value*
	Good	*Moderate*	*Poor*	
Age group				
Young-old (60–69 years)	44.0	40.4	15.5	
Old-old (70–79 years)	29.6	54.3	16.0	12.97***
Oldest-old (80+ years)	15.4	53.8	30.8	
Number of sons				
No son	43.8	43.8	12.5	1.81
One or more sons	36.0	45.8	18.2	
Number of daughters				
No daughter	41.5	40.0	18.5	0.95
One or more daughters	36.6	46.8	16.6	
Work status				
Currently working	48.3	36.8	14.9	5.94**
Currently not working	33.3	48.8	17.8	
Type of family				
Single	46.2	30.8	23.1	
Nuclear family	37.0	47.5	15.5	4.18
Joint family	34.4	47.5	18.0	
Economic dependency				
Economically dependent	31.0	50.6	18.4	7.82**
Economically not dependent	46.8	38.1	15.1	
Health status				
Very good/good	78.3	18.3	3.3	
Fair	36.3	46.0	17.7	64.77***
Poor/very poor	18.1	58.6	23.3	

Significance level given as **: P<0.05, ***: P<0. 01.

Economic dependency of the elderly widows has shown significant impact on health adjustment. Elderly widows who were economically not dependent on others were having good health adjustment. Elderly widows who are economically independent can spend their money on their health care. Whenever they need health assistance, they can seek on their own. Health status has been found to be a significant factor for health adjustment of elderly widows.

Psychological Health Status of Elderly Widows

To measure the level of depression or psychological condition of elderly widows, Geriatric Depression Scale (GDS) was used in this study. This scale is a self-reported 30-item inventory with simple 'Yes/No' answers designed specifically to identify depression among elderly. The time frame for this scale is last one month. This scale has 84 per cent sensitivity and 95 per cent specificity at a cut-off point of 11. It has also high test-retest reliability and internal consistency (Yesavage et al., 1982). GDS can be used among healthy people, physically ill individuals, and those who are suffering from a moderate degree of cognitive impairment. Answers to the questions are simple, can be used in both hospital and community population and administering the instrument does not always require a trained interviewer.

For the purpose of the present study, 24 items have been selected from the 30-item GDS scale. This scale was earlier used in the western settings. In order to adapt the scale to the Indian situation, certain questions were excluded from the scale as it may not be relevant in the Indian context. Certain questions were modified as per the requirement and the scale was finalized. The total score is calculated by totalling one point counted for each depression answer. The score given for the construction of the present scale:

- Score of 0–8: no depression or normal
- Score 9–17: mild depression
- Score over 18: severe depression.

After checking the reliability with alpha values (0.6516), the composite index was computed. Answers to the questions are simple, can be used in both hospital and community population and administering the instrument does not always require a trained interviewer (Table 6.13). (Annexure D – for details of GDS).

Table 6.13

Depression among Elderly Widows

Depression	*Percentage*	*Frequency*
No depression	22.3	67
Mild depression	46.7	140
Severe depression	31.0	93
Cronbach's Alpha Value	**0.6516**	

Based on the GDS, it was found that around 47 per cent of the elderly widows were having mild depression and 31 per cent were severely depressed. While discussing with the government medical officer of study village, he said – *'Loneliness and depression are common among the elderly widows. Depression leads to more serious health problems'*.

The level of depression among the elderly widows according to background characteristics are presented in Table 6.14. Loss of a spouse at any age has a very significant impact on the psychological status of an individual. Around 46 per cent of young-old widows were having mild depression. In the old-old age groups, 48 per cent elderly widows were having mild depression. Among the oldest-old widows, around 35 per cent were severely depressed and 46 per cent were having mild depression.

Elderly widows having a son had an impact on their psychological health. The analysis shows that among elderly widows having no sons, around 35 per cent are severely depressed. However, elderly widows having one or more sons, around 30 per cent are severely depressed. Chi-square test was performed to show the association between background variables and level of depression among the elderly widows. Number of sons, work status, type of family, economic dependency, and receiving pension were emerged as significant factors at 10 per cent level of significance. Current health status was significant at 1 per cent level of significance.

Work status of the elderly widows shows that those who were presently working, slightly less than half (48%) of them were having mild depression whereas, among those who were not working, 32 per cent were severely depressed. This may be because those who are working can engage their time with work or they are going out for meeting people. Those who are not working have a lot of free time and they are spending most of the time sitting idle at home which makes them more dependent on others and feel depressed.

Table 6.14

Per cent Distribution of Elderly Widows by Level of Depression according to Background Characteristics

Background Characteristics	*Depression Level*			
	No Depression	*Mild Depression*	*Severe Depression*	*X^2 Value*
Age group				
Young-old (60–69 years)	23.3	46.1	30.6	
Old-old (70–79 years)	21.0	48.1	30.9	0.43
Oldest-old (80+ years)	19.2	46.2	34.6	
Number of sons				
No son	12.5	51.6	35.9	4.58*
One or more sons	25.0	45.3	29.7	
Work status				
Currently working	23.0	48.0	28.7	0.29*
Currently not working	22.1	46.0	31.9	
Type of family				
Single	20.5	43.6	35.9	
Nuclear family	22.0	46.0	32.0	1.70*
Joint family	24.6	50.8	24.6	
Economic dependency				
Economically dependent	23.6	47.7	28.7	1.06*
Economically not dependent	20.6	45.2	34.1	
Current health status				
Very good/good	46.7	40.0	13.3	
Fair	18.5	52.4	29.0	33.04***
Poor/very poor	13.8	44.0	42.2	
Pension status				
Receiving pension	27.7.	44.6	27.7	5.06*
Do not receive pension	17.1	48.7	34.2	
Duration of widowhood				
Less than five years	18.6	42.4	39.0	
6–10 years	32.0	40.0	28.0	5.24
More than 11 years	20.9	49.7	29.3	

Significance level given as *: P<0.1, ***: P<0. 01.

Regarding the type of family of elderly widows, it was found that of those who were living alone, around 35 per cent were severely depressed compared to those who were staying in joint families. *'It is the responsibility of family members to take care of the elderly and widows. But many family members never worried for the mental peace of their elderly parent' (Key informant interview with a government doctor of the study village).* Economically dependent elderly widows are more severely depressed than that of economically independent.

Health status is also associated with the level of depression. Elderly widows who perceive their health as very good or good, 47 per cent of them reported as normal psychological condition. However, those who were having poor or very poor health condition, only 13 per cent were reported as normal. Findings also show that those who do not receive pension, depression level is high compared to those who receive.

As the duration of widowhood increased, the proportion of severely depressed elderly widows decreased. If the duration of widowhood was less than five years, 39 per cent of elderly widows were in severe depression and 42 per cent were moderately depressed. When the duration of widowhood was more than 11 years, around one-fifth (20.9%) were in normal mental health and 28 per cent were severely depressed. In the initial years of widowhood, women face many problems such as economic difficulties and social problems, but as years go by they cope with the situations and find their way to live with that. They start adjusting themselves to the new situation.

Living Arrangements and Level of Depression among Elderly Widows

It is said that the presence of family members is very important as they provide emotional as well as instrumental support to elderly. So in this study, an attempt was made to understand the level of depression according to the living arrangements of elderly widows and the findings are presented in Table 6.15. Of the elderly widows who were living alone, around 36 per cent were severely depressed. of the elderly widows living with unmarried children, only 15 per cent were not depressed. Elderly widows who are living with their married children and other relatives, 46 per cent were moderately depressed and 30 per cent were severely depressed.

Table 6.15

Level of Depression among Elderly Widows by Living Arrangements

Living Arrangements	*Depression Level*			
	No depression	*Mild depression*	*Severe depression*	*X^2 Value*
Living alone	20.5	43.6	35.9	
Living with unmarried children	15.9	54.5	29.5	2.2*
Living with married children and other relatives	24.0	45.6	30.4	

Significance level given as *: P<0.01.

Leisure Time Activities of Elderly Widows

To understand how elderly widows spend their time, several questions related to their leisure time activities were asked in the survey. It was observed (Table 6.16) that nearly half of the elderly widows spent their leisure time for sleeping. However, 63 per cent of the respondents reported that they prefer to sit idle. Thirty-six per cent spend their leisure time in talking with others and around 22 per cent also play with their grandchildren. Eleven per cent of them watch television in their free time while around 7 per cent engage in religious activities such as prayers or visiting temples.

Table 6.16

Proportion of Elderly Widows by Leisure Time Activities

Leisure Time Activities	*%*	*Number*
Sitting idle	63.0	189
Sleeping	53.0	159
Talking with others	36.0	108
Playing with grandchildren	21.7	65
Watching television	10.7	32
Doing prayers/visiting temples	6.7	20
Reading	0.7	2
Other activities*	3.0	9

* making leaf plate, puff rice, stitching cloths, taking care of animals.

Note: Percentage may add up to more than 100 because of multiple responses.

Substance Use among Elderly Widows

Questions were also asked to the elderly widows about the type of substance use. Survey (Table 6.17) revealed that 42 per cent of elderly widows consume tobacco (*khainee*) and 24 per cent consume *pan*. Eleven per cent said that they consume '*tari*' (locally made alcohol) whereas 7 per cent consume bottled alcohol. '*Gutka*' is being consumed by around 6 per cent of the respondents.

Table 6.17

Proportion of Elderly Widows by Substance Use

Substance Use	%	*Number*
Tobacco	42.0	126
Gutka	6.0	18
Pan	24.3	73
Alcohol	7.3	22
Tari (locally brewed alcohol)	11.3	34
Other*	1.0	3

* smoking bidi, hukka etc.

Note: Percentage may add up to more than 100 because of multiple responses.

Majority of elderly widows who consume tobacco, *gutka* and *pan* reported that they consume almost every day. In case of alcohol (local or foreign liquor) consumption, majority have reported that occasionally they have. Around 8 per cent of elderly widows consume alcohol or *tari* once in a week (Table 6.18).

Table 6.18

Frequency of Substance Use by Elderly Widows

Substance Use#	*Every Day*	*Once in a Week*	*Occasionally*
Tobacco	97.6	1.6	0.8
Gutka	88.9	5.6	5.6
Pan	93.0	5.6	1.4
Alcohol	4.5	9.1	86.4
Tari (locally brewed alcohol)	2.9	8.8	88.2

\# among those who consumes these items.

Summary

In this chapter, an attempt is made to understand the health status and treatment seeking behaviour of elderly widows. For understanding the health status, questions on self-reported health condition, mobility, disability and morbidity were asked. Self-reported health status has been assessed by asking – '*In general, how would you say your health is: (1) very good, (2) good, (3) fair, (4) poor, or (5) very poor'.* Majority of the elderly widows reported their health as fair. About one-tenth felt that their health condition is really very poor. About one-fifth of respondents reported that their health condition is very good or good. Majority among the young-old widows reported their health condition as fair.

As age increases, the health condition deteriorates. Thirty per cent of the oldest-old widows reported that they have very poor health. Only 12 per cent of them have reported very good/good health condition. Of the elderly widows who were engaged in work at the time of the survey, more than half of them have fair health condition. But, of those who were not working, 31 per cent have reported poor health condition.

Family members are prime care-givers, especially in old age. Analysis revealed that elderly widows staying in joint families, less than one-forth have reported very poor health condition. Economic difficulties make elderly widows more vulnerable. Of the elderly widows who are economically fully dependent on others, 13 per cent were reported as having very poor health. Elderly widows who are economically not dependent can spend their money for seeking better health care.

When people are unable to perform the basic physical tasks, they become dependent on others. Understanding the disability among the elderly widows is an important dimension. This is also an indication of decreased functional autonomy and increased demand for long term care. Among the disabled elderly widows, 32 per cent were having more than one disability and more than half suffer from at least one disability. Problem of vision was highest reported followed by difficulty in walking. A sizeable proportion of disabled elderly widows also reported the problem of hearing.

Further, only 13 per cent of disabled elderly widows use physical impairment aid. More than half of the elderly widow stated that their sons are the major source of finance for treatment. One in 10 elderly widows revealed that their family does not bother for their disability at all. Increased age is associated with the increase in disability too. Among all the three categories (young-old, old-old and oldest-old) of elderly widows, problem of vision was more compared to other two problems i.e. hearing and walking. Among the oldest-old widows, more than half had vision problem followed by difficulty in walking.

The morbidity profile among the elderly widows shows that three-fifth reported the prevalence of disease. General weakness, blood pressure, joint pain and gastrointestinal problems were found to be common among elderly widows. Anaemia, paralysis, ulcer, tumour, asthma and filaria were also reported by a sizeable proportion of respondents. Most of the oldest-old widows reported weakness as major health problem. Co-morbidity among the oldest-old widows was more as compared to others. Functional disability was also examined on the basis of curtailments in activities of daily living (ADL). The results suggest that majority of the respondents do not need any help for their basic day-to-day activities. Many elderly widows are not seeking treatment for their health problems because of financial constraint. Those who took treatment for their health problems, on an average spend ₹ 333. Mostly sons or daughters-in-law give money to the elderly widows for seeking treatment.

Health adjustment inventory shows that majority were in moderately health adjusting level and less than one-forth were having poor health adjustment. Age, work status, economic dependency and health status have significant association with the health adjustment among the elderly widows.

Widowhood is the condition which affects psychological health of an individual along with physical health. The geriatric depression scale was administered to understand the depression level among the elderly widows. It was found that majority of the elderly widows have mild depression and 3 out of 10 have severe depression. Economic condition, type of family, health status and living arrangements were significantly associated with the level of depression.

It was observed that nearly half of the elderly widows spent their leisure time for sleeping. About 42 per cent of elderly widows consume tobacco *(khainee)* and around one-fifth consume *pan*. A good number of elderly widows also consume alcohol occasionally.

Overall, the analysis indicated poor health status among most of the respondents. Many were not seeking medical help for their health problems due to financial constraints. Poor economic condition leads to deteriorating health status making many elderly widows vulnerable. Unfortunately, many lack family support when they needed it most.

7

Vulnerability, Coping Mechanism and Support for Elderly Widows

Widowhood has meaning in psychological and social context in which it occurs. If there is anything that a woman abhors in her life, it is the loss of her spouse and becoming a widow (Jamuna et al., 1996). Historically widows are seen as a vulnerable group, with varied positions due to their socio-economic structure (Sheykhi, 2006). Vulnerable groups are those who are unable to protect themselves from abuse, exploitation, or neglect by others (Kim and Geistfield, 2008). Beyond the economic difficulty faced by widows, they often face social and cultural problems. Level of interaction with the family members, friends and neighbours can affect their mental health. One study among the rural widows found that they are more vulnerable to loneliness because of their greater distance from neighbours and services. Further it was observed that poor health, less physical mobility, less satisfaction and frequency of interaction with family and neighbours are often associated with experiencing loneliness among the elderly (Balkwell, 1981). Thus, social support is an important factor which may protect against the potentially injurious effects from stress.

A number of studies have concluded that visits to family members make little difference in the older person's feeling of loneliness or life satisfaction (Arling, 1976). Two reasons have been given for lack of association or negative relationship between family contact and morale. First, elderly people and their children have contrasting interests and thus, they often do not make good companions. Generational differences in socialization and contrasting lifestyles result in a dissimilar set of experiences. Vulnerability has two sides: an external side of risks, shocks and stress to which an individual or household is subject to and an internal side which is defenselessness, meaning a lack of means to cope without damaging loss. The state of widowhood often equates to economic vulnerability for women and further it is associated with the emotional loss and changes in social status. Whereas coping mechanism refers to the set of assets and relationships that allow elderly widows to protect them from a 'bad end' or to recover from a crisis. Coping is an automatic response to overcome difficult situations and coping strategies are things that people do in response to specific stress. Thus, coping is a significant strategy or way that enables the elderly widows to assess their situations, assess the needed skills and face critical distinct life tasks.

Carson et al. (2003) conceptualized three levels of coping which is helpful in overcoming the problematic phases of life:

1. On a biological level, there are immunological defenses and damage repair mechanisms.
2. On a psychological and interpersonal level, there are learned coping patterns, self-defense and support from family and friends.
3. On a socio-cultural level, there are group resources such as religion.

Besides this, social support has been viewed as an important coping resource. Social support refers to the availability of people on whom individuals can rely on and who make them happy. Social network includes people on whom one can rely, friends, neighbours, family members, and people irrespective of sex or age. The social support network is extremely important for elderly widows because their social support play an important role in coping (Sijuwade, 2008).

The development of useful adjustment strategies has been found to be dependent on certain factors like age, religious background, socio-economic status, level of economic dependency, educational attainment, etc. According to Lieberman and Sherman (1989), positive change occurred only among widows who participated actively in social programmes or self-help groups. Several studies on widowhood (Gallagher et al., 1983; Lopata 1996; Momtaz et al., 2009) have found that social network facilitates psychological adjustment following spousal death. This chapter examines the vulnerability of the elderly widows, their coping strategies and the social support they have. The vulnerability of elderly widows has been measured on the basis of their social relationships, change in status after becoming widow, decision-making, etc. In reference to coping strategies, 'Self-Adjustment Inventory' and 'Social Adjustment Inventory' have been employed to understand the situation.

Elderly Widow's Relationship with Neighbours/Friends

In the present study, an attempt has been made to understand the elderly widow's relationship with their friends and neighbours. Table 7.1 reveals that more than half of elderly widows are having a good relationship with their neighbours. Majority of elderly widows stated that they preferred to share their problems with neighbours. However, 66 per cent of the elderly widows do not have any close person with whom they can share their problems. Thirty per cent of the elderly widows share their problems with relatives. More than half of the elderly widows daily spend their time with their friends or neighbours. More than one-fourth (27.5%) of them meet their friends or neighbours weekly. One-fourth of the elderly widows share their problems with close persons who are staying in the same village.

An elderly widow (67 years) stated – *'After the death of my husband, my brother's son has taken all responsibility. He takes care of me like his own mother. My brother and his family are doing everything for me but I do not have anything to give back to them in return'.*

Table 7.1

Distribution of Elderly Widow's Relationship with Neighbours/Friends

	Percentage	*Number*
Relationship with neighbours/friends		
Poor	8.7	26
Average	32.0	96
Good	59.3	178
Any close person/friend for sharing problems		
Yes	34.0	102
No	66.0	198
Person with whom they share their problems*		
Neighbours	68.6	70
Relatives	30.4	31
Friends	1.0	1
Place of stay of the close person*		
Near to house	70.6	72
In the same village, but far from house	26.5	27
In neighbouring villages	2.9	3
How often is time spent with friends*		
Daily	66.7	68
Weekly	27.5	28
Monthly	2.0	2
Occasionally	3.9	3

* Among those who have close persons or friends with whom they share their problems (N = 102).

A question was asked to elderly widows – *'Who takes the decision to meet your friends?'* Majority of elderly widows made their own decision to visit their friends or neighbours. Forty-nine per cent of them often visit the houses of their neighbours or friends. Around 53 per cent of elderly widows said that sometimes their friends or neighbours visit them (Table 7.2).

Table 7.2

Elderly Widows and Interaction with Friends

	%	*Number*
Who takes decision to meet friends?		
Self	99.0	101
Son	1.0	1

Cont'd...

...Cont'd

In general, do you visit your friends?		
Yes	86.3	88
No	13.7	14
Frequency of visit		
Never	13.7	14
Sometimes	37.3	38
Often	49.0	50
Whether friends visit them?		
Yes	97.1	99
No	2.9	3
Frequency of friend's visit		
Never	2.9	3
Sometime	52.9	54
Often	44.1	45
Number of elderly widows	**100.0**	**102**

Interactions with Children

Inter-personal interactions with family members form a very important aspect in anyone's life. Because of need for companionship, it is more significant for the life of elderly women especially after the death of their husbands. The traditional norm in India for an elderly widow is to continue living with children and other kin of her deceased husband or live with one of her sons.

In this study, information on inter-personal interaction of elderly widows with their children was collected. In Table 7.3, percentage of elderly widows by number of their children and the number of children staying with them has been presented. Among the elderly widows who were having one son, in 13 per cent of the cases, the sons are not staying with them. Of the elderly widows having two sons, one-fifth were not staying with sons.

In case of daughters, seven out of 10 daughters are not residing with the widowed mother. As a tradition, daughters once married, carry no financial responsibility for parents but maintain affectionate relationships with them and visit them at regular intervals. Further, information was collected about the place of residence of the children who were not staying with elderly widows. More than half of elderly widows reported that their sons are staying in the same village. In 13 per cent of the cases, sons were staying in a nearby town or city (Table 7.4.).

Table 7.3

Elderly Widows by Number of Children and Children Staying with Them (%)

*Number of Son/s**	*Son/s Staying with Elderly Widows*	
One son	Not staying	12.9
	Yes, staying	87.1
Two sons	Not staying	21.0
	Yes, with one son	43.2
	Yes, with two sons	35.8
Three or more sons	Not staying	15.7
	Yes, with one son	50.0
	Yes, with two sons	10.0
	More than two sons	24.3
*Number of Daughter/s**	*Daughter/s Staying with Elderly Widows*	
One daughter	Not staying	71.0
	Yes, staying	28.8
Two daughters	Not staying	70.0
	Yes, with one daughter	18.1
	Yes, with two daughters	11.1
Three or more daughters	Not staying	71.1
	Yes, with one daughter	15.7
	Yes, with two daughters	8.4
	More than three daughters	5.0

* Information was taken from elderly widows whose children do not stay with them.

Table 7.4

Percentage Distribution of Elderly Widows according to Children's Place of Residence

	%
Son's Place of Residence*	
In same village	52.5
In neighbouring village	40.2
Nearby town/city	13.1
In another district	3.3
In another state/country	4.9
Number of Son/s not Staying with Elderly Widows	*122*

Cont'd...

...Cont'd

Daughter's Place of Residence*	
In same village	11.8
In neighbouring village	56.9
Nearby town/city	24.5
In another district	26.0
In another state/country	22.1
Number of Daughter/s not Staying with Elderly Widows	*204*

Note: Percentage may add up to more than 100 because of multiple responses.
* Information was taken from elderly widows whose children do not stay with them.

In case of daughters, more than 55 per cent of daughters were staying in neighbouring villages. One-fourth of them were staying in another district or nearby town or city. More than one-fifth of daughters were staying in another state. However, 12 per cent of them were staying in the same village where their widowed mother live now.

A comparison between interactions of elderly widows with their son/s and daughter/s has been presented in Table 7.5. One-fourth of elderly widows' sons do not visit them. But majority of daughters visit their elderly mothers. Further probing was done to know the frequency of visit by children. More than half of elderly widows replied that their sons regularly visit them whereas more than two-fifth of daughters visit sometimes or occasionally.

Further, one-fourth of elderly widows said that their sons never communicated with them. However, it is only two per cent in case of daughters. More than half of the daughters communicate with their mothers through telephone. Ninety-six per cent of elderly widows said that their daughters spend enough time with them whenever they visit.

Table 7.5

Percentage Distribution of Elderly Widows by Interactions with Children

Interactions with Son/s	*%*	*Interactions with Daughter/s*	*%*
Son visiting mother		**Daughter visiting mother**	
Yes	74.6	Yes	99.0
No	25.4	No	1.0

Cont'd...

...Cont'd

Frequency of visit by son/s		**Frequency of visit by daughter/s**	
Regularly	57.1	Regularly	20.8
Sometimes	30.8	Sometimes	42.6
Occasionally	16.5	Occasionally	47.0
Frequency of communication by son/s		**Frequency of communication by daughter/s**	
Often	41.0	Often	23.0
Sometimes	21.3	Sometimes	47.5
Occasionally	12.3	Occasionally	27.9
Never	25.4	Never	1.5
Mode of communication		**Mode of communication**	
Telephone	17.6	Telephone	56.9
Letters/Sending person	1.1	Letters/Sending person	1.0
Self-visit	81.3	Self-visit	42.1
Son spending enough time with mother		**Daughter spending enough time with mother**	
Yes	50.8	Yes	95.5
No	49.2	No	4.5
Number of Elderly Widows	**122**	**Number of Elderly Widows**	**204**

Note: Information was collected from elderly widows whose children do not stay with them.

An attempt was made to understand the reasons for not spending enough time by sons with widowed mothers. Figure 7.1 presents the elderly widow's perception on this. More than half of

Figure 7.1

Reasons for not Spending Time by Son/s (%)

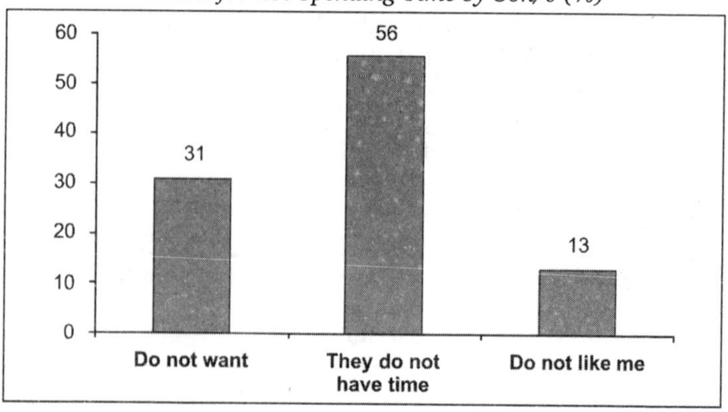

elderly widows perceive that their sons do not have time. Thirty-one per cent of elderly widows stated that their sons do not want to spend time with them as they are busy with their own family. Thirteen per cent felt that their sons do not like them.

In the absence of social security in old age, especially for widows, children are the only means of survival. In general, Indian parents feel that sons will support them in old age. They have more expectations from their sons than their daughters. To know the elderly widows' expectations from their sons, a question was asked – *'what type of care and support one can expect from her son/s'?*

Around 32 per cent of elderly widows expect that their sons should provide food to them. Slightly more than one-fourth of elderly widows have expectations of all kinds of care and support from their sons. Less than 10 per cent of elderly widows expect money from their sons, whereas 14 per cent expect their sons will take care of them in old age (Figure 7.2).

Figure 7.2

Per cent Distribution of Elderly Widows and Expectations from Sons

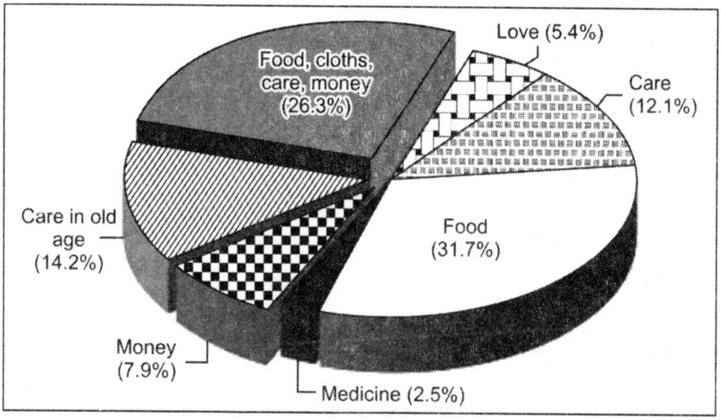

Elderly parents usually expect too much from their sons. Further probing was done to know whether elderly widows are getting expected care and support from their son/s. Thirty-eight per cent of elderly widows are not getting the expected care and support from their sons.

An opinion was sought from elderly widows about the benefit of having a son in their life. A question was asked to all elderly widows who do not have a son – '*Do you think your conditions would have been better, if you had a son*?' More than 80 per cent of elderly widows who do not have a son think that their condition would have been better if they had a son. However, around 16 per cent felt that having a son would have made no difference at all in their living conditions.

Further probing was done to understand which aspects of their life would have been better, if they had a son. About 48 per cent of elderly widows replied that their sons would have taken care of them after husband's death. Around one-fourth of elderly widows said that if they had a son, their economic condition would have been better. Around 4 per cent had revealed that there would not have been any shelter problem for them (Figure 7.3).

Figure 7.3

Elderly Widow's Perception on their Condition would have been Better, if they had a Son

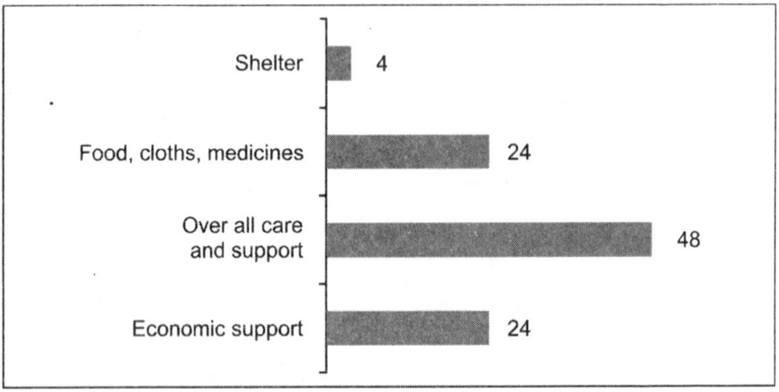

Elderly Widow's Participation in Social and Religious Activities

In the survey, information was gathered about the participation in social and religious activities of elderly widows. Half of the respondents usually participate in family get-together. Half of them do participate in social gatherings like marriage, funeral or any other function. Some of the elderly widows revealed that some people never invite them to social or religious functions.

While interviewing, one elderly widow said – *'I attend marriages in our village. But when the new bride comes to the house, I am not allowed to go there and see her'*. She further mentioned – 'Even *if the new bride comes to our house, I cannot perform any rituals'*.

Table 7.6

Participation in Social and Religious Activities by Elderly Widows

	%	*Number*
Generally do you participate in*		
Wedding	49.7	
Family get-together	50.0	
Funeral	53.3	
Festivals	48.0	
Do you believe in god?	89.0	267
How often do you visit temples?		
Daily	8.3	25
Occasionally	44.0	132
Sometimes	24.3	73
Never	23.3	70
Are you allowed to go out of the village?		
Yes, alone	32.3	97
Yes, with someone	41.0	123
Not allowed	26.7	80
Did you visit/participate in functions outside the village?		
Yes	39.0	117
No	61.0	183
Number of Elderly Widows	**100.0**	**300**

Note: *Percentage may add up to more than 100 because of multiple responses.

Majority of the elderly widows believe in god and 44 per cent of them occasionally visited temples. Around one-fourth of them (24.3%) visited temple sometimes. However, 23 per cent of elderly widows did not visit temples/worship places. Not going to temple is not an indication that they do not believe in god. There are many restrictions in villages on widows' participation in social and religious activities.

It is evident from the analysis that more than half (61%) of elderly widows do not visit or participate in any functions outside village. Around 27 per cent of elderly widows are not allowed to go out of the village to participate in any functions. Forty one per cent of elderly widows are allowed to go out of the village, only when accompanied by someone.

Table 7.7

Elderly Widows Participation in Religious Activities (Before and After Widowhood)

Religious Activities				
Before Widowhood	*%*	*After Widowhood*	*%*	*Paired t-Value*
Never	28.7	Never	35.3	3.354***
Sometimes	36.0	Sometimes	37.3	(0.061– 0.233)
Always	35.3	Always	27.3	

Significance level given as ***: P< 0.01.
Figures in parentheses is 95% confidence interval of the difference.

Table 7.7 presents the participation of elderly widows in religious activities before and after widowhood. Thirty-five per cent of them were attending religious activities before widowhood. But after widowhood, there is a significant decline in the participation of religious activities. This reflected greater isolation and a lack of community identity of the elderly widows. Paired t-test infers there is a significant difference among the elderly widows for attending the religious activities before and after widowhood. Significant positive correlation was found between participation in religious activities before and after widowhood (r=0.54, P< .01).

Decision-Making by Elderly Widows on Various Issues

One way to understand the status of elderly widows is to know their decision-making power on various issues. In this study, an attempt was made to understand the status of elderly widows by their ability to take decisions. Table 7.8 shows that around 48 per cent of elderly widows took their own decisions to visit places outside the village. Forty-two per cent of elderly widows revealed that their sons or daughters-in-law usually take decisions on their behalf regarding their visits outside the village. Around nine per cent of elderly widows stated that they take decisions jointly with someone. On being enquired about the decisions taken regarding the treatment of health problems, 45 per cent of elderly widows stated that their sons or daughters-in-law take decisions about medical treatment.

Table 7.8

Decision Taken by Elderly Widows on Various Issues

Decision Taken on Various Issues	*%*	*Number*
Who takes decisions regarding visiting outside the village?		
Self	47.7	143
Son/Daughter-in-law	41.7	125
Jointly with someone	8.7	26
Others*	2.0	6
Who takes decisions regarding treatment for health problems?		
Self	39.0	117
Son/Daughter-in-law	45.3	136
Jointly with someone	11.7	35
Others*	4.0	12
Type of decisions for which elderly widows were consulted		
All major decisions	22.3	67
Economic decisions	12.3	37
Social decisions	23.7	71
No consultation	41.7	125
Whether advice was sought from elderly widows on decision-making before widowhood?		
Yes	55.3	166
No	44.7	134
Whether advice was sought from elderly widows on decision-making after widowhood?		
Yes	36.0	108
No	64.0	192
Number of Elderly Widows	**100.0**	**300**

Note: *Others includes brother/sister, daughter/son-in-law.

Elderly widows were also asked about the type of decisions in which they were usually consulted by the family members. Forty-two per cent of elderly widows said that they were not consulted while taking decisions. One-fourth (23.7%) of the elderly widows said that during social occasions their family members consult them. Only 12 per cent of elderly widows were consulted on economic matters. One-fourth of them stated that they were consulted on all major decisions taken in the house.

To know the changing status of elderly widows before and after their widowhood, further probing was done to know whether their advice was taken seriously on family matters. More than half (55.3%) of elderly widows reported that their opinions were taken seriously on family matters when their husbands were alive. But after husband's death, majority of the elderly widows were not consulted on any family matters. This shows the changing status of women and reducing decision-making power within their family after widowhood.

Opinion about Status of Elderly Widows

Forty–two per cent of elderly widows felt that their status is low in the village and only one out of seven felt that widows have good status in villages. When asked about the factors responsible for the low status of elderly widows, majority said that economic constraints are the main factors for the poor status of elderly widows in the villages. One-fourth believed that social factors are responsible for the low status of widows.

To examine the status within their own households, a question was asked – *'In your opinion, what is your status within your family?'* The responses were categorized into three – *low, medium and good:* Forty-nine per cent of elderly widows have opined that they have medium status in their households whereas around 32 per cent felt that their status is low. Further, more than half (59.8%) of elderly widows were satisfied with their present status within their families. Forty per cent of them were not satisfied with their status in the house. Majority of elderly widows (59.7%) felt that their status has changed after widowhood. Those who have felt that their status has changed; nearly half of them stated that there is lack of respect from family members after widowhood. One-fourth of them have an opinion that they are not consulted in any family matters after widowhood. Around 12 per cent of the elderly widows also said that after becoming a widow, they have to take permission from their children on all important matters. One in 10 elderly widows were not involved in any family function after widowhood (Table 7.9).

Table 7.9

Self-Perception about Status of Elderly Widows within their Family

Elderly Widows Status Within and Outside Their Family	*%*	*Number*
Status of widows in the village		
Low	42.0	126
Medium	51.0	153
Good	7.0	21
Factors responsible for the low status of widows		
Economic factors	49.5	149
Social factors	23.7	71
Family factors	21.0	63
Religious factors	5.7	17
Elderly widow's status within their own family		
Low	32.3	97
Medium	49.3	148
High	18.3	55
Are you satisfied with your status within your family?		
Yes	59.7	179
No	40.3	121
Whether your status in the family has changed after becoming widow?		
Yes	56.7	170
No	43.3	130
If yes, in which aspects, your status has changed*?		
Lack of respect	47.1	80
Opinion not sought	25.3	43
Need permission for everything	11.8	20
Not involved in family functions	9.4	16
Other reasons#	6.4	11

Note: * among those who said their status has changed after widowhood (N= 170).

other reasons include health-related problems, economic problems, loneliness, etc.

Further, perception about the status of elderly widows within their family according to living arrangements is presented in Table 7.10. Only five per cent of elderly widows who were living alone perceive their status is good within their extended family. Those elderly widows who were living with their married daughter/s, 33 per cent consider their status is low in the household.

Table 7.10

Elderly Widows by their Actual Living Arrangements and Perceived Status within their Family (%)

Actual Living Arrangements	*Perceived Status of Elderly Widows within their Family*			*Number of Elderly Widows*
	Low	*Average*	*Good*	
Living alone	66.7	28.2	5.1	39
Living with unmarried children	27.3	50.0	22.7	44
Living with married son	24.1	53.0	22.9	166
Living with married daughter	33.3	50.0	16.7	18
Living with other relatives	39.4	54.5	6.1	33
Total	**32.3**	**49.3**	**18.3**	**300**

The state of widowhood is exacerbated by conditions of poverty (United Nations, 2001). Around 81 per cent of elderly widows had faced many problems immediately after becoming a widow. More than half of the elderly widows have faced economic problems. Around 35 per cent of elderly widows faced child care problems. Around 14 per cent of elderly widows faced social problems (Table 7.11).

Table 7.11

Type of Problems Faced after Widowhood (%)

Problems Faced	*Never*	*Sometimes*	*Always*
Economic	6.5	26.9	66.5
Housing	57.6	22.4	20.0
Child care	42.0	23.3	34.7
Health care	52.7	31.4	15.9
Food	20.8	33.1	46.1
Social	82.4	13.5	4.1
Others#	95.5	3.3	1.2

Note: Multiple response question.

other problems include problems related to loneliness, emotional problems, etc.

In many rural communities, women were blamed for the death of their husbands. A 65-year-old tribal widow revealed – '*After my husband's death, people said that I am a witch and I only killed my husband. My neighbour one day said that if I want to be alive, then I should not show my face to anyone and stay inside my home*'. Widowhood is still considered as a curse for women in villages. They were exploited and humiliated by villagers for no reasons.

Figure 7.4

Efforts made to Overcome Economic Problems after becoming Widow

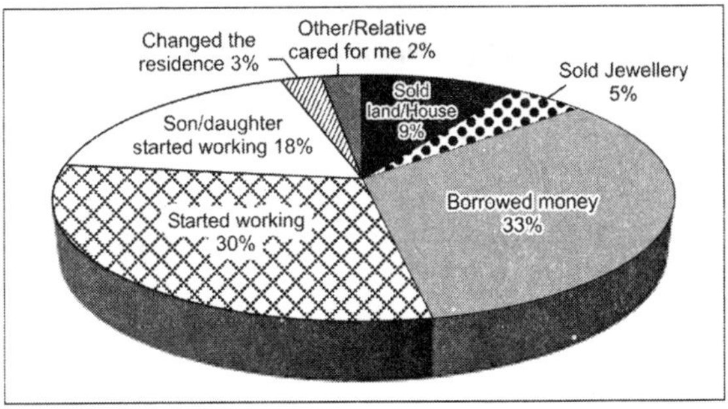

To overcome the immediate problems faced after widowhood, 33 per cent of widows borrowed money and 30 per cent have started working. Nine per cent of elderly widows were forced to sell their houses due to economic crisis experienced after widowhood. Sizable proportion of elderly widows sold their jewellery due to economic necessities after husband's death (Figure 7.4).

After the death of the earning member of the family, it is very difficult to manage the house all alone. Widowhood is a crisis with emotional shock, a drastic change in social status, and often an economic crisis (Bhatt, 2006). The help from the community, family members or from others were a great support during this crisis period. The present study collected information on the help received by elderly widows when they faced problems immediately after becoming a widow. Table 7.12 indicates that more than half of elderly widows do not receive any help from any one. Twenty-eight per cent of elderly widows have received help from the villagers. More than one-fifth (22%) of elderly widows received help from their mother/brothers/sisters whereas one-fifth of them received help from other relatives. Nineteen per cent of elderly widows have got help from their sons. Very few (2.5%) have received help from their brothers-in-law.

An elderly widow narrated the treatment she received from her brother-in-law after her husband's death – *'After the death of my husband, I stayed with my husband's elder brother and his family. They gave me one small room to stay. Sometime I have to beg in the village for my food'.* However, 24 per cent have received care and support from the family.

Table 7.12

Persons Helped Elderly Widows and Type of Help Received

	%	*Number*
Did you receive any help?		
Yes	39.3	118
No	60.7	182
Who helped you? #		
Son	18.6	22
Daughter	8.5	10
Mother/brother/sister	22.0	26
Brother-in-law	2.5	3
Other relatives	20.3	24
Village people	28.0	33
What type of help was received? #		
Money	63.3	75
Food	11.0	13
Shelter	1.7	2
All care and support	23.7	28

based on those elderly widows who received support after husband's death (N= 118)

It is important to examine the elderly widow's continued contact with her husband's family. A question was posed – *'How is your relationship now with members of your husband's family?'* Thirty per cent of the elderly widows were not having any contact with their husband's family (Figure 7.5). *'Vidhava hone ke baad, koi apne sasural mein kaise rahega? (After widowhood, how can you stay at your in-laws house?)'* – as stated by an 82-year-old widow.

Figure 7.5

Elderly Widows Relationship with Husband's Family

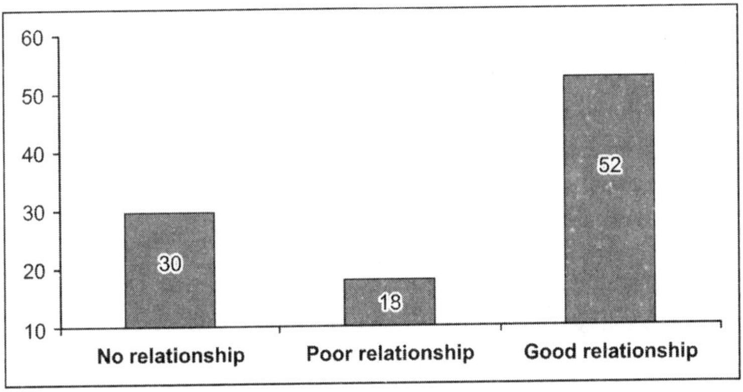

Did elderly widows get the same respect and care from her husband's family before and after widowhood? The question was – *'Before and after the death of your husband, were you treated with respect by your husband's family?'* More than half of elderly widows reported that they were not treated with respect by husband's family after widowhood.

There is an increase in percentage of elderly widows who were treated badly by husband's family. Twenty-two per cent of the elderly widows were looked after badly by their husband's family before widowhood. But after widowhood, it has increased up to 45 per cent, indicating a significant difference in the behaviour of husband's family before and after widowhood (Table 7.13).

Table 7.13

Treatment of Elderly Widows by In-laws Before and After Widowhood

Treatment of Elderly Widows by Husband's Family	*Before Widowhood*	*After Widowhood*	*Paired t-Value*
Bad	22.3	45.3	8.938***
Indifferent	28.0	23.7	(0.325 –0.508)
Good	49.7	31.0	

Significance level given as ***: P<0.01

Figures in parentheses is 95% confidence interval of the difference.

Emotional Deprivation

The widowed are emotionally deprived and do not have any intimate person to share their problems. To examine this, a series of statements were asked to the elderly widows. They were requested to mention either *'yes'* or *'no'* to each of the statement. To understand the emotional deprivation among elderly widows, a composite index was computed using the seven statements canvassed. After checking the reliability with alpha values (0.8649), the composite index has been computed. The total score ranging from 0 to 7 indicates the emotional deprivation among them. On the basis of total scores and the mean value, the score has been categorized into three – *'normal'*, *'low'* (score ranging from 1–2) and *'high'* deprivation (score 3 and above).

On the basis of the computed composite index, 46 per cent of elderly widows felt high level of deprivation at emotional level (Figure 7.6). Further, Table 7.14 shows that more than half of the oldest-old widows are at high derivation level on emotional issues. Oldest-old widows usually stay at home most of the time and nobody is there to talk to them. High emotional deprivation was found among the elderly widows who were living alone. Further, it was observed that economic dependency and emotional deprivation are significantly co-related.

Figure 7.6

Percentage of Elderly Widows Feel Emotionally Deprived by their Family Members

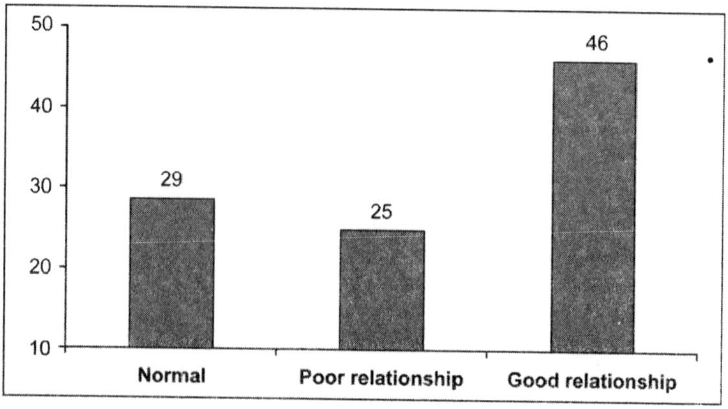

Table 7.14

Emotional Deprivation among Elderly Widows according to Selected Background Characteristics

Selected Characteristics	*Level of Emotional Deprivation*			X^2 *Value*
	Normal	*Low*	*High*	
Age Group				
Young-old (60–69 years)	30.1	23.3	46.6	
Old-old (70–79 years)	25.9	30.9	43.2	2.53
Oldest-old (80+ years)	26.9	19.2	53.8	
Type of family				
Single	10.3	23.1	66.7	
Nuclear family	31.0	23.5	45.5	11.41
Joint family	32.8	31.1	36.1	
Economic dependency				
Economically dependent	35.1	30.5	34.5	23.39***
Economically not dependent	19.8	17.5	62.7	

Significance level given as ***: P<0.01

Here, an attempt was made to understand whether elderly widows are satisfied with their status in the family. Table 7.15 indicates that majority of elderly widows whose status within their family is low are not satisfied. But, among those who are having better status in the family, around 90 per cent are satisfied with their present status. Half of the economically dependent elderly widows revealed that they are not at all satisfied with their status within their own family.

Table 7.15

Elderly Widows Satisfaction with the Perceived Status within Family and Level of Economic Dependency (%)

Perceived Status of Elderly Widows Within their Family	*Satisfied With Status within Family*		
	Yes	*No*	*Number*
Low	18.6	81.4	97
Average	75.0	25.0	148
High	90.9	9.1	55
Level of Economic Dependency			
Fully dependent	68.6	31.4	121
Partial dependent	64.2	35.8	53
Independent	49.2	50.8	126

Loneliness is a common problem among widows. Women feel lonely more than men and the loss of the spouse accentuates these differences. The death of a partner means an end to daily conversation and also an end to many shared activities in which the spouse was the driving force. Death of husband can affect the relationship between family members. Loneliness is a kind of status which emerges due to setback in the family cohesiveness. It also indicates the disorganization in personality among elderly in particular (Yadava, 2011).

Table 7.16

Distribution of Elderly Widows on their Feeling of Loneliness, according to Selected Characteristics

Selected Characteristics	*Feeling of Elderly Widows about Loneliness*				X^2 *Value*
	Never	*Sometimes*	*Often*	*Total*	
Age group					
Young-old (60–69 years)	33.2	42.0	24.9	193	3.1
Old-old (70–79 years)	25.9	46.9	27.2	81	
Oldest-old (80+ years)	34.6	30.8	34.6	26	
Type of family					
Single	12.8	23.1	64.1	39	38.3***
Nuclear	31.0	45.5	23.5	200	(d.f = 4)
Joint	44.3	44.3	11.5	61	
Living arrangements					
Living alone	12.8	23.1	64.1	39	42.4***
Living with unmarried children	22.7	43.2	34.1	44	(d.f = 6)
Living with married children	37.9	44.8	17.2	203	
Living with other relatives	14.3	57.1	28.6	14	
Level of economic dependency					
Fully dependent	33.1	51.2	15.7	121	32.1***
Partial dependent	37.7	50.9	11.3	53	(d.f = 4)
Not dependent	27.0	30.2	42.9	126	
Perceived status of elderly widows within their family					
Low	13.4	33.0	53.6	97	61.4***
Average	36.5	48.0	15.5	148	(d.f=4)
High	49.1	43.6	7.3	55	

Significance level given as ***: P<0.01, (d.f is degree of freedom)

A question was asked in the survey – *'How frequently do you feel lonely, even when you are with members of your family?'* The responses to this question were grouped into three categories – *never, sometimes and often*. Table 7.16 shows the distribution of feeling loneliness among elderly widows according to selected background characteristics.

One-fourth of young-old widows and 35 per cent of oldest-old widows often felt lonely. According to the type of family, more than three-fifth of (64%) elderly widows who stay alone often felt lonely. The type of family was found significantly associated with the extent of loneliness.

The study shows that there is significant association between living arrangements and loneliness among elderly widows. Thirty-four per cent of elderly widows living with their unmarried children often feel lonely. Those who are living with married children may be busy with their grandchildren. Forty-three per cent who are economically not dependent on others often feel lonely. However, 49 per cent of elderly widows who consider having high status within their family never felt lonely.

A question was asked to elderly widows – *'Who took care of you after the death of your husband?'* In half of the cases, son or daughter-in-law took care of them after the death of their husbands. Around 15 per cent of elderly widows managed themselves.

Table 7.17

Distribution of Elderly Widows by Care-Takers after Husband's Death

Care Takers after Husband's Death	*%*	*Number*
Self	15.7	47
Son/daughter-in-law	49.0	147
Brother-in-law	13.7	41
Daughter/son-in-law	5.7	17
Brother/sister	8.7	26
Others*	7.2	22
Total	**100.0**	**300**

Note: *others includes grandchildren, mother, father, uncle and other relatives.

Self-Adjustment of Elderly Widows

A self-adjustment inventory has been used in this study to understand how elderly widows are adjusting with their life problems. To assess the self-adjustment among the elderly widows, a set of questions were asked. The statements were framed in such a way that it could be answered either as *'yes'* or *'no'*. A set of questions – 'Do you think that *you are much better than many other women of your age? Do you have any hobby to engage your time?'* – were asked to understand the adjustment among the elderly widows. The questions in the self-adjustment inventory were modified to suit Indian rural situation. One point is given to each answer which shows the adjustment among the elderly widows. After checking for the reliability test, the alpha value comes to 0.5368. The scale of self-adjustment has been categorized as 0–4 points: *'Poor'*, 5–8 points: *'Average'* and 9 and above points: *'Good'*.

Figure 7.7

Self-Adjustment of Elderly Widows (%)

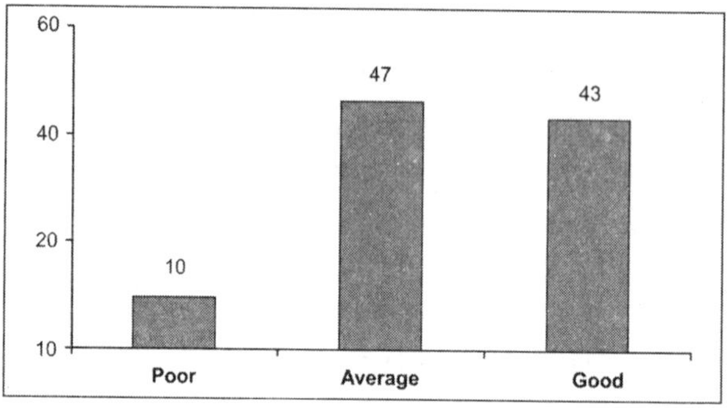

Figure 7.7 shows that 43 per cent of the elderly widows were found to be 'good' in self-adjustment, whereas 10 per cent are 'poor' in self-adjustment of their life problems.

The level of self-adjustment among the elderly widows has been shown by the background characteristics in Table 7.18. Young-old widows were performing better in self-adjustment. Poor self-adjustment was reported more among the old-old widows compared to young-old widows (8.3%). Work status has shown positive and significant correlation with self-adjustment of elderly widows. More than half (51.7%) of the working elderly widows are 'good' at self-adjustment. Majority among the elderly widows who live alone have poor levels of self-adjustment. One in 10 elderly widows from nuclear families were poorly self-adjusting. Elderly widows residing in joint families have relatively less difficulty in self-adjustment. This may be due to the presence of many family members, including children and grand-children, who usually take care of the requirements of the elderly.

Significant association has been observed between perceived health status and self-adjustment among elderly widows. It is also observed that elderly widows who were at low level of emotional deprivation were having 'good' self-adjustment.

Table 7.18

Self-Adjustment of Elderly Widows by Selected Background Characteristics

Selected Characteristics	*Self-adjustment*				X^2 *Value*
	Poor	*Average*	*Good*	*Total Number*	
Age Group					
Young-old (60–69 years)	8.3	45.6	46.1	193	
Old-old (70–79 years)	13.6	42.0	44.4	81	8.7
Oldest-old (80+ years)	11.5	69.2	19.2	26	
Work Status					
Currently working	5.7	42.5	51.7	87	4.6*
Currently not working	11.7	48.4	39.9	213	
Type of Family					
Single	15.4	51.3	33.3	39	
Nuclear family	10.0	44.5	45.5	200	3.5
Joint family	6.6	50.8	42.6	61	
Economic Dependency					
Economically dependent	10.3	44.8	44.8	174	0.5
Economically not dependent	9.5	49.2	41.3	126	
Health Status					
Very good/good	1.7	36.7	61.7	60	
Fair	8.9	40.3	50.8	124	28.1***
Poor/very poor	15.5	58.6	25.9	116	
Emotional Deprivation					
Normal	1.2	36.0	62.8	86	
Low deprivation	4.0	44.0	52.0	75	41.8***
High deprivation	18.7	54.7	26.6	139	
Total	**10.0**	**46.7**	**43.3**	**300**	

Significance level given as *: P<0.1, **: P<0.05, ***: P<0.01.

Social Vulnerability among Elderly Widows

Societies differ considerably in culture and social systems. The status of a widow varies considerably among the societies. In India, many Hindu women regard widowhood as a punishment given to them by god for the crimes committed in their previous birth. Moreover, widowhood is a life-event that removes not only a person's support system but also reduces the size of informal support network at the same time (O'Bryant, 1988).

In the primary survey, an attempt was made to understand whether the elderly widows are getting due respect from the younger generations. Thirty-one per cent of them felt that younger generation is not paying them the respect they really deserve. This opinion is mainly due to the respondents' comparison of the situation at two points in their life time– when they were young and when they were old. They naturally tend to compare the extent of respect they have shown to their elders and the type of respect that they now receive from the youngsters.

Why there is a shift in paying respect towards elders? More than three-fifth (65%) of elderly widows said that the young people do not like the old people. Around one-fifth of them felt that youngsters are busy in their own work and have no time for the aged (Figure 7.8).

Figure 7.8

Reasons for Young Generation's Attitudes Towards Older Persons (%)

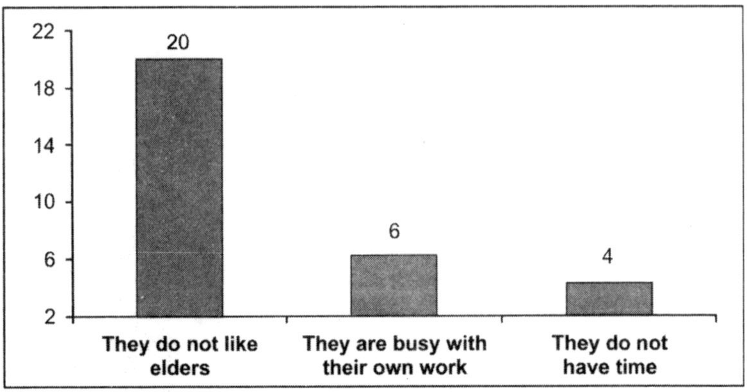

Further, a question was asked – *'Do you think widows are not properly treated in your village?'* More than half of the elderly widows consider that widows are properly treated by the villagers. Most of the elderly widows (60.7%) blame their own fate for the present pathetic condition. Around two-fifth have blamed their own family members for the problems. More than one-fourth of elderly widows have an opinion that village community and widows themselves are responsible for their miseries. Slightly less than one-fourth of elderly widows blamed the government and traditions existing in our society for this helpless situation and poor status of widows.

Figure 7.9

Elderly Widow's Opinion about who should be Blamed for their Pathetic Condition (%)

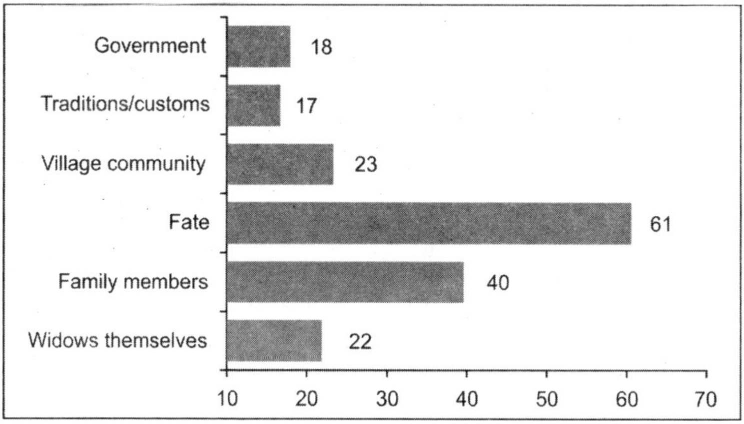

Note: Multiple response question

What can be done to improve the status of widows? More than half (57%) of elderly widows stated that widows should be economically supported (through regular pensions). One-fourth of elderly widows said that they should get free health service. Twelve per cent of elderly widows felt that a widow welfare committee should monitor their problems. Many have submitted the required documents to Block Office for the pension. But when they go there, either nobody responds to them or declare that they are not eligible for a pension.

Demand for an old age home was reported by only three per cent of elderly widows. Around one per cent of them wanted free travel facility and other facilities like free distribution of food, etc. (Figure 7.10). However, most of the elderly widows need financial support to improve their living conditions.

Figure 7.10

What can be done to Improve the Life Situation of Widows?

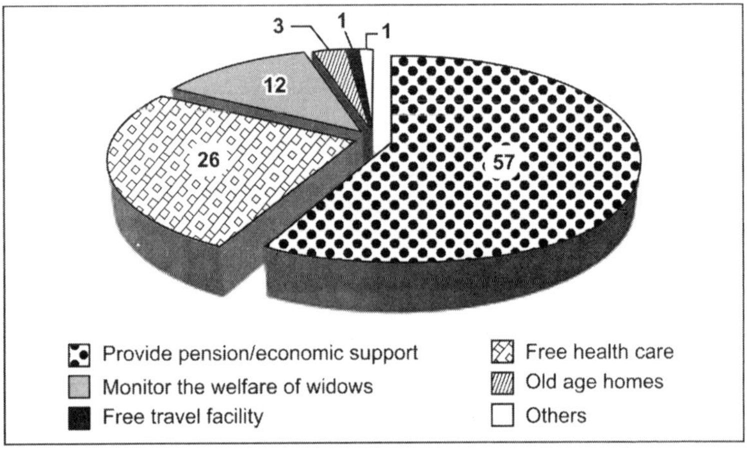

Note: others include food, job, etc.

Social-Adjustment Inventory of Elderly Widows

Social adjustment refers to the subjective satisfaction with relationships or performance in social roles (Shapiro and Keyes, 2008). In spite of social exclusion, widows try to adjust with the society in which they live. To understand the social adjustment among the elderly widows, social adjustment inventory was employed. A set of questions consisting of 16 items were asked to the elderly widows and one point has been given to each answer which shows the social adjustment among them. Out of 16 items, two items have been dropped as these two were not showing significant correlation with the other variables. So, 14 items were used for the computation of composite index of social adjustment. The reliability with alpha values comes to 0.6315. The score has been categorized into three – *'low'* (0–4 score), *'medium'* (5–9 score) and *'high'* (10 and above score) levels of social adjustment.

Fifty two per cent of elderly widows were found to have good social adjustment, according to this study (Figure 7.11).

Figure 7.11

Social-Adjustment of Elderly Widows (%)

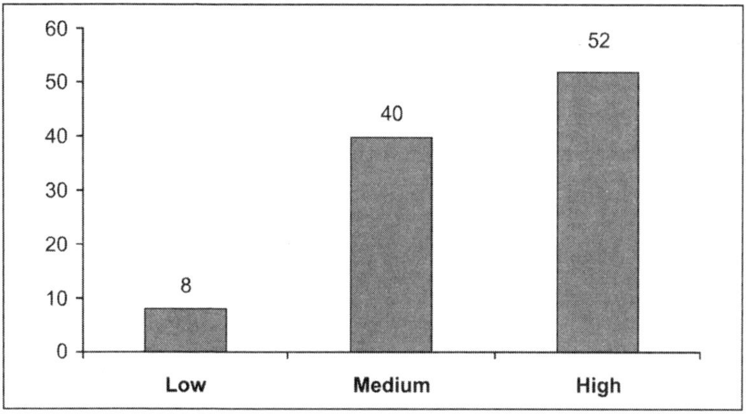

Table 7.19 shows the social adjustment among elderly widows by background characteristics. No significant correlation was observed between the work status and social adjustment of elderly widows.

Table 7.19

Social-Adjustment Inventory among Elderly Widows by Selected Background Characteristics

Selected Characteristics	*Social-Adjustment*				X^2 *Value*
	Low	*Medium*	*High*	*Total Number*	
Age Group					
Young-old (60–69 years)	10.4	38.3	51.3	193	
Old-old (70–79 years)	3.7	40.7	55.6	81	3.8
Oldest-old (80+ years)	7.7	46.2	46.2	26	
Work Status					
Currently working	6.9	37.9	55.2	87	0.6
Currently not working	8.9	40.4	50.7	213	

Cont'd...

...Cont'd

Type of Family					
Single	15.4	33.3	51.3	39	
Nuclear family	8.0	41.0	51.0	200	3.9
Joint family	4.9	39.3	55.7	61	
Economic Dependency					
Economically dependent	4.0	43.7	52.3	174	10.9
Economically not dependent	14.3	34.1	51.6	126	
Health Status					
Very good/good	6.7	35.0	58.3	60	
Fair	8.1	33.9	58.1	124	7.4*
Poor/very poor	9.5	48.3	42.2	116	
Emotional Deprivation					
Normal	2.3	29.1	68.6	86	
Low deprivation	1.3	37.3	61.3	75	34.3***
High deprivation	15.8	47.5	36.7	139	
Total	**8.3**	**39.7**	**52.0**	**300**	

Significance level given as *: P<0.1, ***: P<0.01.

Fifteen per cent of elderly widows living alone were showing low social adjustment as compared to four per cent who live in joint families. Fourteen per cent of economically independent elderly widows were at low social adjustment. Those who were having good or very good health conditions, more than half of them were indicating high level of social-adjustment. Emotional deprivation among elderly widows has shown significant co-relation with their social-adjustment.

Awareness of Widow Remarriage Act and Opinion Regarding Widow Remarriage

The Hindu Widow Remarriage Act was passed on 26 July 1856, permitting widow remarriage to be performed in the same way as the first marriage. The Act has two main provisions. First, widow remarriage would be legally valid and the offspring would be legal. Second, the widow would forfeit all claims to wealth and/or financial support inherited through her earlier marriage.

In the present study, a question was asked to the elderly widows about the awareness of Widow Remarriage Act and their opinion regarding remarriage. The survey indicated that more than half of the elderly widows in the sample are not aware of Widow Remarriage Act. More than 60 per cent of elderly widows, who were aware of Widow Remarriage Act, supported the widow remarriage (Figure 7.12). However, even now many women believe that widows should not go for a second marriage.

Figure 7.12

Awareness about Widow Remarriage Act and Opinion about Remarriage

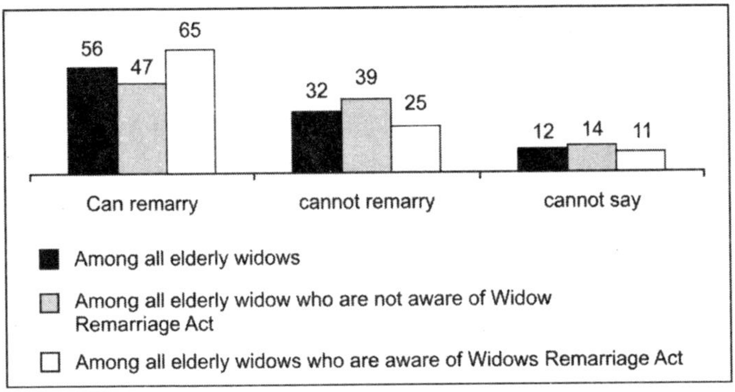

Though remarriage is not forbidden but there are several reasons due to which widows do not want to remarry. Reasons given by the elderly widows are presented in Figure 7.13.

Figure 7.13

Reasons for not Remarrying

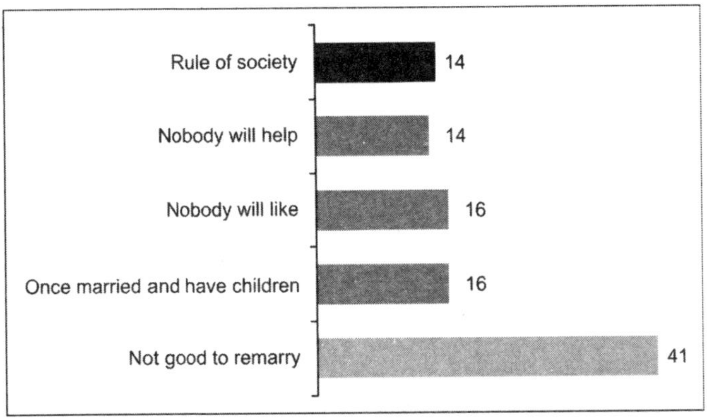

Majority of the elderly widows stated that it is not good to remarry after the death of one's husband. However, 14 per cent have mentioned that this is the rule of the society that a widow cannot marry again after her husband's death. Sixteen per cent of elderly widows cited – *'If a woman is once married and is having children from her first husband, then she should not remarry'*. Few elderly widows have also stated that in case widows opt for remarriage, family and community may not support her.

While talking about the attitudes regarding the widow remarriage, a 60 year-old Muslim widow stated – *'If a woman becomes a widow at a very young age and does not have any children, then it is better for her to get married again. Otherwise, it is not good to remarry because who will take care of her children. It is not sure that her second husband and his family will accept the children from the first husband'*. Further she mentioned – *'I was interested in remarriage, but because of my three children, I decided not to marry again'*. The negative attitude towards remarriage is so strong that even today many people believe that it will not get social and religious sanction.

Figure 7.14

Elderly Widow's Opinion about their Remarriage after Widowhood

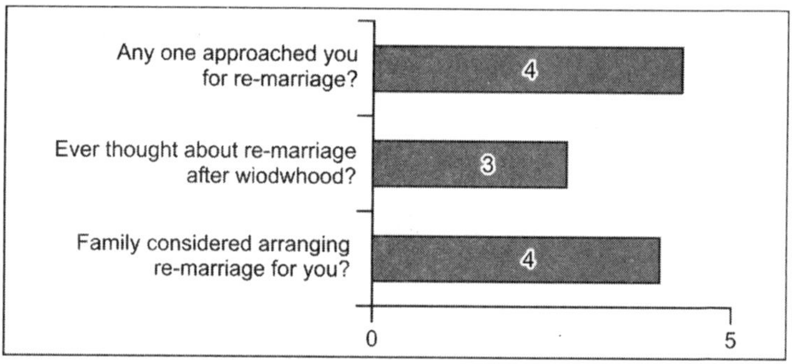

During the interviews, the information was gathered about widow remarriage of respondents by asking questions like *'Did at any time your family consider for arranging a remarriage for you? At any time, did any one approach you with a marriage proposal? Did you reject any second marriage proposal?'* Only 4 per cent of the elderly widows revealed that their family members considered for arranging remarriage for them. Less than 3 per cent of elderly widows have ever thought about remarriage after becoming a widow and around 4 per cent also received marriage proposals. These findings show that widow remarriage is not common and not acceptable to the society in rural areas (Figure 7.14).

Family and Community Reactions on Widow Remarriage

In a traditional Indian society, a widow is not allowed to remarry or it is not socially encouraged. Widow remarriage is not still socially approved in spite of its legal sanction. To understand the family and community reactions on this issue, a question was asked to the elderly widows – *'In case you had opted for remarriage, what you think about the reactions of your family or community?'* Family and community reactions as perceived by the elderly widows have been presented in Table 7.20.

Table 7.20

Family and Community Reactions towards Widow Remarriage

Family Reactions	%	*Community Reactions*	%
Expel from house	21.3	Expel from village	25.0
Family never accepts it	40.6	Community will not accept it	20.7
Family would beat me	9.3	Community may accept	19.0
Not in our culture	9.3	Do not know the reaction	13.0
Family will be happy	11.0	Not allowed in community	7.0
Not good to go for remarriage	8.0	Not good	15.0
Number of Elderly Widows	**300**	**Number of Elderly Widows**	**300**

Majority of elderly widows perceive that their family would have never accepted the remarriage if they had opted for it. Slightly more than one-fourth of elderly widows stated that in case of remarriage, family would throw her out of the house. Eleven per cent of elderly widows felt that their family would have been happy, if they had opted for remarriage.

While discussing about the possible community reactions towards widow remarriage, slightly less than one-fifth (19%) of elderly widows felt that widow remarriage will be acceptable to the community. However, one-fifth of elderly widows also felt that, if they had opted for remarriage after widowhood, community would have boycotted them.

Knowledge about Rights of Elderly and Widows

On 15 August 1995, the Government of India had announced the National Social Assistance Scheme (NSAS) which talks about the public assistance in old age. In 1999, the Government of India announced another social scheme called 'Annapurna' for its elderly destitute (Rajan and Mathew, 2008). Although there are many social assistance programmes in India, but only few poor or illiterate people knew about these schemes.

This study made an attempt to understand the knowledge of respondents about the rights for the elderly citizens and widows. Table 7.21 shows that more than half of elderly widows do not have any knowledge about the rights for elderly or widows. Majority (78.7%) among them, who have some knowledge, only heard about the pension schemes or Indira Awas Yojana.

Table 7.21

Per cent Distribution of Elderly Widows who are Aware about Welfare Schemes for the Elderly or Widows

	%	*Number*
Knowledge of any welfare schemes for elderly or widows		
Yes	45.3	136
No	54.7	164
Type of schemes known to the elderly widows#		
Pension/Indira Awas Yojana	78.7	107
Free food	15.4	21
Free health check-up	3.7	5
Free travel facility	2.2	3
Source of information #		
Women of same age	36.0	49
Village people	61.0	83
Village head (Sarpanch)	2.9	4

Note: #based on elderly widows who knew about the rights of elderly or widows (N= 136).

Further, it was asked – *'Have you heard about old age homes? Do you know about any old age home?'* Sixty-five per cent of the elderly widows in the sample had never heard about old age homes. After explaining about the purpose of old age homes, 60 per cent still did not prefer to stay in an old age home (Table 7.22).

Table 7.22

Elderly Widow's Knowledge about Old Age Homes

	%
Ever heard about old age home	
Yes	35.0
No	65.0
Know any old age home	
Yes	19.0
No	81.0
Prefer to stay in old age home	
Yes	40.3
No	59.7
Number of Elderly Widows	**300**

Figure 7.15

Reasons given by Elderly Widows for not Staying in Old Age Homes (%)

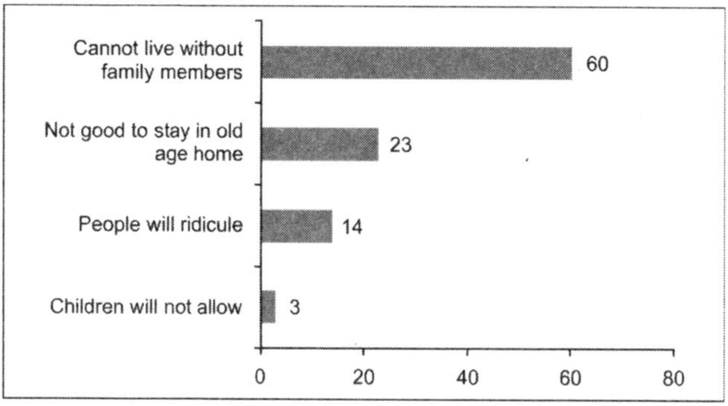

When asked about the reasons (Figure 7.15) for not opting for an old age home, most of them said that they cannot live without family members. Slightly more than one-fifth (22.9%) of them stated that it is not good to stay in an old age home, if they have children. While interviewing, one elderly widow said – *'Most people in the old age homes are there because their family members*

do not want to take care of them. If I stay in an old age home, then villagers will think that my family members are against me'.

The traditional norms and values of the Indian society have always emphasized on respect and care for the aged. The aged members are normally taken care of by the family members. In recent times, due to breaking of joint family system, a large number of old parents is not maintained by their children. Consequently, the elders are now exposed to emotional neglect and lack of physical and financial support. To ensure the maintenance of aged parents by their children as a legal right, 'The Maintenance and Welfare of Parents and Senior Citizen's Bill' was passed by the Indian Parliament in 2007. The main objective of the bill was to provide for more effective provisions for maintenance and welfare of parents and senior citizens and to make the maintenance of the parents mandatory on children. 'Maintenance' includes provision for food, clothing, residence and medical attendance and treatment. Although the bill was passed long back, still this act is not yet implemented in all states of India. In the state of Jharkhand, it is not implemented.

Only 14 per cent of the elderly widows in the sample knew about this Act. But they do not know the name of the Act. Few have some knowledge that if children are not taking care of their parents, then parents can go to court for justice. Further, it was asked – *'In case a situation arises, will you go to court against your child (ren) to claim maintenance?'* Majority (72%) of the elderly widows stated that they will not go to court against their child (ren). In the words of an elderly widow (67 years) – *'Lardka jitana bhi bura ho jay, lekin maa to nahi hogi na (Son can be bad, but mother never do so)'.* Many elderly widows said that all depends on one's luck. According to another respondent – *'May be I am not fortunate enough. I lost my husband early. My sons do not want to look after me. My daughters-in-law hate me. I must have done something wrong in my previous life'* (Widow aged 75 years).

Mistreatment or Abuse Experienced by Elderly Widows of Study Areas

'Life has become a hell for me. Who will take care of a woman when she is widowed?' (A widow aged 64 years). Many elderly women,

particularly widows, are exposed to abuse and mistreatment within their own families. It was found that female elderly, particularly widows, are more vulnerable to elder abuse and neglect in Indian families (Sebastian and Sekher, 2011).

American Psychological Association (2004) defines elder abuse as – 'It is the infliction of physical, emotional, or psychological harm on an older adult. It also can take the form of financial exploitation or intentional or unintentional neglect of an older adult by the caregiver'. To know the abuse or mistreatment experienced by the elderly widows, a question was asked– '*Do you try to avoid some members of this family?*' followed by another question – '*Are you afraid of anybody with whom you are currently staying?*' This question was asked to the respondents when no one else was present there at the time of interview.

Figure 7.16

Mistreatment Experienced by Elderly Widows within Family (%)

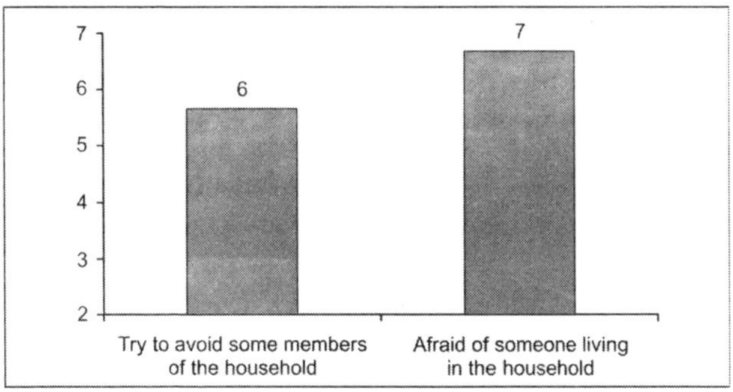

Seven per cent of elderly widows in the sample were afraid of someone in their own family (Figure 7.16). Being widowed and aged, they are more vulnerable to abuse and neglect. Around five per cent of elderly widows reported that they were physically harmed by someone in the household.

An elderly widow (83 years) living alone narrated her experience – '*My daughter-in-law always quarrels with me. My son and daughter-in-law are not taking care of me. My neighbours help me in doing my work*'. In her own words – '*Isi din ko dekhane ke liye itana kast karke bete to aadmee banaya, par mujhe kya pata that ki beta aisa ho jayega, (I have taken all pains to bring up my son. But for whom I was doing all the hard work all these years, now treats me like this!)'*

Figure 7.17

Neglect Experienced by Elderly Widows (%)

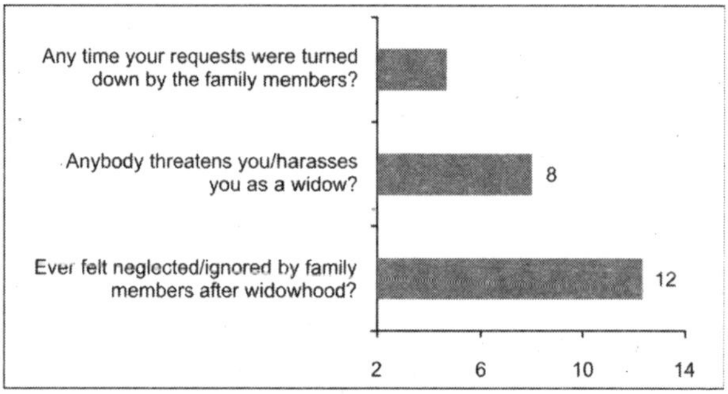

Many elderly widows are considered as a burden by family members. Young children do not like elderly members interfering in their personal matters. Figure 7.17 shows that 12 per cent of elderly widows from the study villages felt neglected or ignored by their own family membres. Around 8 per cent of elderly widows revealed that they are being threatened by someone and 5 per cent have said that their requests for help were mostly ignored by family members.

Summary

This chapter examines the vulnerability, coping mechanism and support available to the elderly widows. Elderly widows suffer multiple problems attributable to gender, widowhood and old age. An attempt has been made here to explain the types of deprivations elderly widows face and their adjustments with the problems. The study has shown that elderly widows face problems within their house and within the community. Widowhood is a life event which removes not only the older person's closest person but also reduces the size of the informal social network. Although most elderly widows have good relationships with their neighbours, but not many elderly widows have someone intimate enough to share their problems.

The likelihood of receiving help for an elderly widow not only depends upon the socio-economic characteristics but also the presence of the children. Many elderly widows do not have the support of their sons. In many cases, sons are staying in the same village but in a different house. Most of the daughters are staying in the neighbouring villages. Sons visit their elderly mothers regularly. One-fourth of the sons never communicate with their elderly mother. More than half of the respondents feel that their son(s) does not spend enough time with them. More than two-fifth of elderly widows believe that their conditions would have been better if they had a son. Around one-fourth of elderly widows revealed that their sons would have supported them economically.

Parents expect something from their children. Majority of the respondents stated that they expect their sons should provide food to them in old age. Less than 10 per cent of elderly widows have expectation of receiving financial support from their sons. However, some of the elderly widows stated that their expectations from their son(s) are not fulfilled.

Elderly widows participate in social and religious functions in the family and in the community. Few elderly widows revealed that they do not come forward to perform any rituals in marriage ceremony. More than two-fifth of elderly widows visit temples occasionally. A significant difference was found among the elderly widows attending the religious activities before and after widowhood.

Elderly widows are usually given a role in taking decisions on social matters. But in major issues like financial matters, elderly widows were not consulted. Forty-two per cent of elderly widows are not having any say over family matters. More than two-fifth of elderly widows felt that they have low social status in the village. The economic constraints are the main factors for the low status of the widows.

Six per cent of elderly widows believe that religious factors are also responsible for the poor status of widows in the village. More than half of elderly widows felt that their status in the family has changed after the death of their husbands. They are getting comparatively less respect from other family members.

Eighty-one per cent of elderly widows faced problems immediately after becoming widow. They have faced economic difficulties, followed by housing problems. Three-fifth of elderly widows have not received any help from any one after the death of their husbands. For 19 per cent of elderly widows, their son(s) helped them after the death of their husbands.

With regard to the relationship with the husband's family, half of the elderly widows continue to have good relations with their in-laws. However, three out of 10 elderly widows do not have any contact with their husband's family. Some of the elderly widows have also stated that husband's family did not treat them properly.

Oldest-old widows are physically and economically more dependent on others which makes them more vulnerable and emotionally deprived. Loneliness among the elderly widows was reported as a major problem; particularly in later in life (after 80+ years). More than two-fifth of elderly widows living alone often feel lonely.

According to the present study, 10 per cent of elderly widows have 'poor' self-adjustment. Work status, health condition and emotional deprivation have significant association with self-adjustment. Age, type of family, and economic dependency has not shown any significant association with self-adjustment.

Joint family system is slowly breaking down even in rural areas. The influence of modern lifestyles on younger generation and the changing attitudes towards the elderly are two important aspects. Thirty-one per cent of elderly widows felt that young people do not really respect them. More than two-fifth of elderly widows think that they are not being treated properly in the village. Majority blame their fate for the pathetic condition. Around 17 per cent of elderly widows blamed the prevailing customs for their miserable conditions.

More than half of the elderly widows were not aware about the Widow Remarriage Act. Majority have said that after the death of husband, it is not good to remarry. Few elderly widows believe that as a rule of the society, a woman cannot remarry after becoming a widow. Some of them said that a widow can remarry under the condition that she is not having a child from the first marriage and she is young. However, very few elderly widows have ever thought of remarriage. Majority of the elderly widows felt that family would have never accepted their second marriage. Around one-fifth of elderly widows perceived that they would have been thrown out of their houses, if they had opted for a remarriage.

More than half of the elderly widows in the sample do not have any knowledge about the benefits available for the elderly or widows. More than three-fourth of them are aware about the pension schemes or Indira Awas Yojana. More than half of the elderly widows have not even heard about old age homes. Few elderly widows also mentioned that one can stay in an old age home, if she does not have any one to support her.

Eighty-six per cent of elderly widows do not have any knowledge about the new 'Maintenance Act'. Further, majority have said that they will not go to court against their own children to claim maintenance.

Few elderly widows of the study area were experiencing mistreatment or abuse within the family. Around 7 per cent of elderly widows were afraid of someone with whom they were currently residing. Around 5 per cent of elderly widows experienced physical harassment from family members. Twelve per cent of elderly widows felt neglected or ignored by family members. In general, elderly widows face many problems and multiple discriminations. This varies from economic difficulties, lack of physical help and social stigma. Since they have no other option, many silently suffer this neglect.

8

Summary, Conclusions and Recommendations

Summary

Widowhood places women in a disadvantaged position, particularly in their old age. Widows are the most vulnerable segment of the elderly population in rural India. Widow's condition is directly related to lack of access to economic resources including land ownership, inheritance of property, lack of support system and their marginalization and exclusion from the decision-making process. Elderly widows face several problems such as lack of status within family as well as in society, loneliness, poor economic status, lack of social recognition, depression, health problems, lack of care from the family members, etc. However, very few studies have examined the conditions of elderly widows.

The main objectives of the present study are: (1) to examine the living arrangements of elderly widows in rural areas, (2) to study the socio-economic status and level of dependency of elderly widows, (3) to study the health status (physical and psychological) and the treatment seeking behaviour of elderly widows, and (4) to understand the extent of vulnerability and the coping mechanism of elderly widows within the family and in the community.

To fulfil the above stated objectives, the present study utilizes both primary and secondary data. Census of India and two rounds of NSSO (52nd and 60th Rounds) data were analysed to understand the scenario of elderly in general and elderly widows in particular at the national level. The primary data was collected from two blocks of East Singhbhum district of Jharkhand state. The selected district has highest proportion of elderly in the state, according to 2001 Census. Primary data consists of information from interviews with 300 elderly widows. In order to complete the targeted sample size, 12 villages from the two blocks were visited. The data collection was carried out from March to June 2010. Pre-tested, semi-structured interview schedules were used for collecting the quantitative data from the identified households having elderly widows. Two different sets of interview schedules – Household Schedule and Individual Schedule – were administered. Apart from this, case studies and key informant interviews were conducted to gather qualitative information on specific issues related to elderly widows.

Macro level scenario of elderly widows shows that they are mostly economically dependent on others. Majority of elderly widows are living with their children but few of them are forced to live alone. Significant proportion of elderly widows in India faces problems in meeting the requirements such as – food, clothing and medicine. Findings also indicated that an elderly widow's participation in social and religious functions is low.

Very few elderly widows have reported their current health status as excellent or very good. The reported diseases among the elderly widows are higher than the aged in general. Locomotor disability among the elderly widows is high compared to disability of vision and of hearing.

Majority of the surveyed households were Hindus, followed by Sarna and Muslims; majority were Scheduled Tribes. More than half of the surveyed households have no ownership of land. Less than one-fourth of the households lived in *pucca* houses. Dry leaf/wood/coal/charcoal/dung cakes were the major sources of fuel for cooking for majority of the households. Seven out of 10 households do not have access to toilet facility. More than half of the households reported that their main source of drinking water is public piped water/hand pump/covered well. Half of the surveyed households have BPL cards. Many surveyed elderly widows were receiving widow pension of ₹ 200 per month.

Study has shown that 13 per cent of elderly widows were living alone at the time of the survey. When preferred living arrangements were analysed, it was found that among those elderly widows who were living alone, about one-fourth preferred to live with their married sons.

As it is important to know the living arrangements of the elderly, it is also important to know their satisfaction with the current living conditions. More than one-third of elderly widows living alone stated their living arrangements as 'uncomfortable'.

Analysis suggests that most elderly widows living with their married children (son/daughter) or grandchildren are comfortable with their present living conditions as compared to those who were living alone. Number of children is one of the important determining factors in deciding the living arrangements of elderly widows. As the number of sons or daughters increases, more elderly widows reported their living condition as 'comfortable'. This may be because they are getting the support, care, love and respect from sons or daughters, and this fulfils most of their needs in old age.

More than two-fifth of elderly widows have changed their place of residence after their husband's death, as nobody from their family wanted to keep them. Most of the elderly widows in the sample were economically dependent on others. Majority of elderly widows do not have any savings. More than half of those who were receiving pension stated that the pension money is not enough to fulfil their basic requirements. Regarding the ownership of land and house, majority of elderly widows neither own a house nor land.

To understand the health status of elderly widows of the study areas, questions on self-reported health condition, mobility, disability and morbidity were asked. Self-reported health status has been assessed by asking – *'In general, how would you say your health is: (1) very good, (2) good, (3) fair, (4) poor, or (5) very poor'*. Study has shown that majority of elderly widows reported their health as fair.

Inability to perform the basic physical tasks makes people dependent. Physical dependency of elderly widows decreases their functional autonomy. Among the disabled elderly widows, more than half suffers from at least one disability and 32 per cent were having more than one disability. The problem of vision was more prevalent, followed by difficulty in walking among the elderly widows of study area. Only 13 per cent of the disabled elderly widows use any aid for physical impairment.

Most of the oldest-old widows reported weakness as major health problem. Co-morbidity among the oldest-old widows is more as compared to other age groups. Overall, the analysis indicated poor health status among most of the respondents. More importantly, many were not seeking medical help for their health problems due to financial constraints. Poor economic condition leads to deteriorating health, making many elderly widows vulnerable. Unfortunately, many lack family support when they needed it most.

Geriatric Depression Scale (GDS) was administered to understand the psychological condition of the elderly widows. This is a 30-item scale employed to find out the level of depression among the elderly. According to GDS, 47 per cent of the elderly widows interviewed were having mild depression and 31 per cent were suffering from severe depression.

Further, an attempt was made to explain the nature of deprivations elderly widows usually face and their adjustments and coping mechanism. The study has shown that they face many problems within their house and within the community. Although most of the elderly widows have good relationship with their neighbours, but not many have someone intimate enough to share their problems with. The likelihood of receiving help for an elderly widow not only depends upon the socio-economic characteristics, but also on the number of children they have. Many elderly widows believe that their conditions would have been better if they had a son. However, some of the elderly widows also felt that having a son would not have made any difference in their living conditions.

To measure the extent of emotional deprivation among the elderly widows, a composite index was computed using seven statements. The computed index has shown that elderly widows suffer from emotional high deprivation.

Elderly widows are usually given a role in family decision-making on social matters. But in major issues like financial matters, elderly widows were mostly not consulted. More than half of elderly widows felt that their status in the family has deteriorated after the death of their husbands. Elderly widows opined that their views were taken seriously on family matters when their husbands were alive. But after husband's death, majority of them were not consulted in any family matters. Thirty-two per cent of elderly widows perceive that they have low status in their households. The economic constraints are the main factors for the low status as stated by elderly widows. Many elderly widows, who were living with their married daughter/s, consider their status as low in the household.

Elderly widows of the surveyed villages face many problems immediately after becoming a widow. Three-fifth of elderly widows have not received any type of help from any one after the death of their husbands. Some of them also stated that their husband's family did not treat them properly. Few among them revealed that now they do not have any contact with their husband's family. Many times widows in the villages were blamed for the death of their husbands.

To understand how elderly widows are adjusting with their life problems, self-adjustment inventory was employed in this study. The questions in the self-adjustment inventory were modified to suit Indian rural situation. According to this, 43 per cent of the elderly widows were found to be 'good' in self-adjustment, whereas 10 per cent were 'poor' in self-adjustment. Family plays an important role in the self-adjustment of elderly widows.

Around one-fifth of elderly widows interviewed felt that youngsters are busy in their own work and have no time for the aged. Most of the elderly widows blame their own fate for the present pathetic condition. However, many have an opinion that village community and the widows themselves are responsible for the situation. On the other hand, few elderly widows blamed the government and the existing traditions in the rural society for their helpless situation.

To understand the social adjustment among the elderly widows, a social adjustment inventory was employed in this study. More than half of the elderly widows found to have 'good' social adjustment. Elderly widows living alone were showing low social adjustment as compared to those who live in joint families. Health conditions and emotional deprivation among the elderly widows have shown significant co-relation with their social-adjustment.

More than half of the elderly widows are not aware of Widow Remarriage Act. Majority of the elderly widows stated that it is not good to remarry after the death of the husband. Majority of them perceived that their family would have never accepted the remarriage, if they had opted for it.

Many elderly widows in the sample do not have any knowledge about the benefits/schemes available for elderly or widows. More than half of the elderly widows of the study area have not even heard about old age homes. When asked about the 'Maintenance and Welfare of Parents and Senior Citizen's Bill' which was passed by the Indian Parliament in 2007, only 14 per cent of the elderly widows in the sample knew about this Act. However, majority of the elderly widows stated that they will not go to court against their own child/(ren), if the situation arises.

Few elderly widows of the study area are experiencing mistreatment or abuse within the family. In general, elderly widows face many problems and discrimination. This varies from economic difficulties, lack of physical help and social stigma. Since they have no other option, many silently suffer this neglect. High level of illiteracy, lack of remunerative occupation, as well as negligible awareness about legal and economic rights makes them more vulnerable to neglect and abuse.

Conclusions

In conclusion, the present study revealed that elderly widows face discrimination both at the household and at the community levels which varies from economic, physical to emotional needs. Being aged as well as widowed they do not have intimate persons with whom they can share their problems. Though family members are taking care of the elderly widows in most cases, they also face neglect and abuse in some households. Many elderly widows felt lonely after the death of their husbands. Along with poverty and economic constraints, mistreatment and neglect by the family members makes them further vulnerable. Most of them silently cope up with this situation.

Recommendations

The main dimensions which impact the well-being of elderly widows are economic, health and social aspects. There are other aspects like education, status and respect, community activities, and societal attitudes which also indirectly influence their quality of life in old age.

In light of the findings emerging out of the present study, welfare measures for the elderly, especially for the widows, need to be developed. Considering the low levels of literacy among them, their primary occupation in the unorganized sector, poor financial security in terms of possession of assets, property and income, their overall low standard of living which denies them basic amenities of daily living, appropriate welfare programmes need to be designed.

Due to loneliness, many of the mental health problems such as feeling of insecurity, depression, etc. are reported. Loneliness many times leads to depression and isolation of widowed women. So, there should be some support system, especially for those who are suffering from physical or mental illness. Further due to ageing, there are also physical health problems and lack of medical treatment due to financial constraints. There is a need of schemes to look after the health of elderly widows. In addition, in view of increasing disease burden and disabilities affecting the elderly, as well as their lifestyle patterns which further threaten their health, the governmental health services need to be equipped in terms of infrastructure and manpower training to address these special health needs of the elderly.

Sometimes widows are discouraged from taking part in auspicious ceremonies and social activities. Even today, widows in rural areas are accused of being responsible for the death of their husbands. Based on the realization that widowhood is generally stressful for women, it is hereby recommended that massive and intensive campaign should be mounted to sensitize people on the need to stop all forms of abuse and discrimination associated with widowhood. Widows need to be provided with functional education capable of emancipating them from the stress and tensions of widowhood.

The family as a fundamental unit of society has to be strengthened as a support system for the provision of care and protection for older persons, particularly for elderly widows. The emotional, social, physical and economic support provided by the family was indispensable and cannot be replaced by any other institution. For this reason, attention should be given to promote co-residence through housing policies and financial incentives for those households where the elderly are family members. Special attention should be given to vulnerable older persons such as the widows, the childless, the disabled and the sick, whose families are unable to support them and those who are destitutes. Financial security should be provided to low income families having elderly or widows. There is also a need to develop counselling services for both widows and their family members.

The Indian elderly widows become over dependent on family members for economic and emotional purposes. This condition is to be changed by giving them more authority and power. If the widowed women are willing to work, some type of occupation should be provided to make them feel useful to the society and at the same time, earn some money for themselves.

Policies and programmes should ensure that older persons have a reasonable and adequate living environment. For this, incentives should be given to facilitate appropriate housing schemes for elderly widows who live alone either by choice or by circumstances. Besides, there should be an evaluation of the various ongoing schemes of the government to establish the usefulness of these provisions to the welfare of the elderly and widows.

Limitations of the Study

The present study highlights the socio-economic and demographic characteristics of elderly widows of rural areas only. In the present study, mainly the elderly widow's experiences and opinions were considered. The perspective of other family members of the household was not taken into account. Due to operational reasons, the elderly widows who refused to be interviewed or not in a healthy condition to be interviewed were left out of the sample. Though all efforts were made to gather the information on sensitive issues such as mistreatment and abuse, it is also possible that many elderly widows were reluctant to reveal the extent and nature of mistreatment they experienced both within families and in the village society.

Scope for Future Research

With increasing number of aged in India, the problems of elderly will be manifold. The present study has tried to understand the living conditions and problems of elderly widows of rural areas. A comparative study can be done between elderly widows and widowers to investigate and compare the situation among them. It is difficult to cope up with the problems especially after widowhood, so there is a need to examine the different coping mechanisms adopted by the widows and widowers.

Appendix A

Case Studies of Elderly Widows

Case Study 1

Mrs A is a widow aged 75 years. She got married at the age of 12 to a man of 18 years of age. They were staying in village Patpur and working as vegetable vendors. They have five daughters and one son. They both worked hard to support their children and to get them married. When her first daughter got married they were really happy. But 10 days after the marriage, daughter returned back home because her husband was previously married to another woman, which was not known to others. Mrs A's second daughter got married in a nearby village but after some time her husband sent her back saying that she is suffering from many diseases. Other daughters and son also got married and were staying separately. When Mrs A's husband passed away due to sudden illness, she was only 40 years old. After that she was staying with her only son. But after son's marriage, his behaviour changed drastically and he showed very little interest in looking after his old mother.

Mrs A owns 6 bigha of land which she inherited from her father. Her son was worried that his mother will give all the property to the two daughters who are separated from their husbands. He started misbehaving with mother, including physically harassing her. The daughter-in-law was not giving enough food and would not talk to her deliberately. On many occasions, daughter-in-law misbehaved with her and this has led to conflict between mother and son.

Later, she sold her land to build a house in a nearby village and is now living with her two daughters. Mrs A complained to village elders on many occasions about the misbehaviour of her son and daughter-in-law. Each time her son assured everybody that he and his wife will behave properly and take care of his mother. But things continued the same way. Mrs A's two daughters, who are staying with her now, are engaged in some works for earning a livelihood. One has a *'pan'* shop and another makes envelops and sells them in the market. Mrs A also sells puffed rice in the market to earn a small income. Now she is happy living with her daughters and does not want to stay with her son. However, she has no bad feeling towards her son and daughter-in-law. In her own words – *'Ladka jitana bhi bura ho jay, lekin maa to nahi hogi na. (Son can be bad, but mother can never do so).'*

However, she believes her daughters saved her life when she was facing difficulties and abuse. In her own words – *'Beti hai to abhi main hun, nahi to kahi bheek mangati hoti (I have daughters; otherwise I would have been now begging on streets)'.* She also realized that daughters are as valuable as sons. She has seen sons taking care of their parents so well in her neighbourhood. But Mrs A was not lucky enough. Her son only wanted parental property, not his mother. Though she did everything possible to make her son's life comfortable, the reward she got was only abuse and ill-treatment. According to her:

> May be I am not fortunate enough. I lost my husband early. My son did not want to look after me. My daughter-in-law hates me. I must have done something wrong in my previous life.

I can see the helplessness of an elderly widow in Mrs A. When I bid good-bye to her after a long chat, she was almost crying. With tears in her eyes and voice choking with emotions, she said – *'I do not want to live any more. I pray to god to take me back as early as possible. I do not want to suffer more and become a burden on anyone'.* She has no interest to live. She has no idea what is in store for her. Life has given her many painful experiences. She expected too much from her son but ended up with great disappointment.

Case Study 2

Mrs B is a widow of 60 years of age having two sons and one daughter. She became a widow after 16 years of her marriage. Her husband was a vendor of toys. Her husband died in a bus accident. When she became a widow suddenly, her children were too young. Her mother-in-law and sister-in-law were also staying in the same house. She was doing all the household works and her mother-in-law never allowed her sister-in-law to help her in the household work. After her husband's death, the situation became more pathetic. She started selling bangles in nearby villages to earn some money. Somehow she has managed the burden of her children's education. The two sons studied up to only class fifth and seventh. Her mother-in-law and sister-in-law never took care of children. She was feeling so insecure for her daughter and so sent the daughter to her brother's place for education. There she studied up to class tenth.

Her brother helped her at the time of her husband's death by giving some money but on many occasions, he refused to give her more money. Her brother suggested her to go for remarriage but she refused by saying that she is ready to work and take care of her children on her own. She sold the silver jewelry which she got during her marriage and repaired the house and also arranged the marriage of her sister-in-law. Now, her two sons are working as a casual labourers and she is also working as a maid servant in a nearby house. She also sells bangles for an extra income.

She said – '*When a woman becomes a widow, it is very difficult to manage everything alone and it becomes more difficult when family members do not support*'.

Her mother-in-law expired a few years back. Now she is staying with her two sons. Sometimes her sister-in-law comes to meet her. But sister-in-law comes home to ask for money and to quarrel with her. Mrs B never thought that she cannot manage her problems. She stated – '*It was difficult for me to manage a family after the death of my husband, but god was kind enough*'. Her sons are also doing some work to manage the family and providing economic support to her. She is searching a suitable boy for her daughter, but being alone it is a difficult task for her. Although her brother promised to help in her daughter's marriage, she was not comfortable to depend on him. Now her sons are earning money and she is also working. She said – '*God should show mercy to every woman, especially to widows*'. When her husband expired, her life was so miserable and she considered of going back to her brother's house. But if she would have gone, then they would have forced her for a second marriage. For the sake of her children, she had decided not to marry again.

When I was interviewing her, she started crying. '*Ek aurat ka jab pati mar jata hai to ghar ke hi log saath nahi dete to government ya kissi aur se kya umeed karenge, (when a woman becomes widow, and her family members do not support, how can I expect anything from the government or help from some other people?)*'.

When I asked her about her opinion on remarriage, she said – '*If a woman becomes a widow at a very young age and does not have any children, then it is better for her to get married again*'. Further she said – '*If in-laws are supportive, then there is no need to marry again*'. She believes that she has taken the right decision in her life and because of that her children are doing well now. Finally she said – '*I want to see my children live happily. That is my only wish now*'.

Case Study 3

Mrs C is a widow aged 76 years. She got married when she was 16. At the age of 44 years, she became a widow. She has one son and three daughters. When her husband died, her younger daughter was only two years old. She got 85 bighas of land from her father at the time of marriage. Her husband was managing a shop and also cultivating their land. She sold her land for the treatment of her husband.

After his death, her condition became very pathetic. Somehow she managed for some years. Her three daughters and son got married. After two years of her son's marriage, daughter-in-law started quarrelling with her. She never gives her enough food. She was forced to work as a sweeper for 8–10 years. Her two daughters were staying in nearby villages and one was in the same village. One day her son and daughter-in-law told her to leave their house. This was a shock to Mrs C. Then she started living with her daughter in the same village. Her daughter and son-in-law have a small shop.

She said – *'If you have money, then people will ask about you. But if you have nothing, then nobody will even come to see you'*. She continued – *'Every parent hopes that their son will take care of them in old age. It is better to have a daughter rather than a son. If I do not have a daughter, then I will be begging somewhere now'.*

After the death of her husband, she suffered a lot. She said – *'I did not know for whom I am working so hard, my son will throw me out when I really needed his help'*. She still expects love and care from her son. *'What I am expecting from my son may be I will get in my next birth'.* Her son and daughter-in-law stay in the same village but they never come to see her even during her ill health. Mrs C. had no option but to stay with her daughter, though it is not common in villages to live with son-in-law. *'When I was young, I never thought that one day I will be living in my son-in-law's house. What can I do?'*

I could see the frustration and hopelessness in a widow's life. All her hopes were shattered when her son and daughter-in-law started abusing her. She never had happiness and peace of mind. 'Well, we expect many good things, but we get many bad things in life' – at the fag end of her life, this widow has become philosophical.

Case Study 4

Mrs D is now 72 years old. She got married when she was just nine years to a man of 20 years. He was an agricultural labourer. They never had any children. Due to financial problems, they could not consult doctors for his health problems and he passed away two years ago. Now, she is staying with her husband's elder brother. They have given her one small room. They never give her sufficient food. She cannot see properly, due to cataract. *'When my husband was alive, at least I was getting food two times. Now I have to beg the villagers for food. Sometimes, I have to go to bed without dinner'.* Further she mentioned – *'I wish, I would have had a son or daughter so that they would have taken care of me after my husband's death. At least I need not to go to every house pleading for food. When I fall sick, nobody is here to look after me. I have applied for pension many times, but I am not getting it. I have visited the Block Office on many occasions but nobody there listens to me. Now I have no hope from them'.* She has no idea why pension was denied to her.

At the time of her husband's death, village people helped her with some money. When I was interviewing her, she said – *'I came to know that a girl from the city has come to our village to talk with the old women. Can you do something for me? Why am I not getting a pension? Will you help me to find out?'*

She said, *'I want to stay with my husband's elder brother, but they are not ready to support me. They have given me one room but I want them to take care of me'.* She believes that pension money will help her to buy whatever she wants. *'My brother-in-law is not helping me nowadays. When I need any help, he simply refuses. But in front of villagers, he acts like taking care of me. Everyone in this village knows my condition'.*

She wants to visit 'Varanasi' but she is does not have money for that. Further, she said, *'If my husband was alive today, then I would not have faced any problem'.* When I asked her about old age homes, she had no idea about it. When I explained her about the old age homes she was ready to go there. She said– *'Although I am staying with my brother-in-law, I am staying here as a neglected person in this house. It is better to live in an old age home, at least there will be some people whom I can talk with. I will get love and care from people living there'.* Now she is mentally prepared to go to any old age home.

After completing the interview when I said good-bye to her, she was in tears. She accompanied me for some time and made a request, with lot of hesitation, *'Can you find out an old age home for me where I can live rest of my life? I am sure; god will be kind to you if you are kind to an old widow'.*

Case Study 5

Mrs M is a 67-year-old widow, who belongs to a Scheduled Caste family. She was working as a cleaner (sweeper). Her husband retired as an electrician from a government water pump station. They do not have any children. Suddenly one day her husband passed away. After his death, nobody was there to look after her. Now she is staying with her brother's son who is a rickshaw puller. He tries to help her in all possible ways with his limited income. She gets care and love and is very happy living here.

During interview, she said – *'I am having one problem. I am not getting my husband's pension and because of this, I feel that I am a burden on my brother's family. My brother and his family are doing everything for me but I do not have anything to give to them in return. Sometimes I feel very lonely'. She adds, 'Agar mera ek beta hota to achha hota. Mera dekh-bhal karta. (If I had a son, then he would have taken care of me after my husband's death.)'*

Since, she is illiterate and do not have any documents, so could not get the pension of her husband. Her brother is a rickshaw puller and do not have time to go to the town office enquiring about pension. She does not have any problem in staying with her brother's family but if she gets the pension money, then she will be able to contribute to the family's day-to-day expenditure.

She is also worried about her future. *'Now my health is fine and I can manage everything on my own. But after some time, what will happen? Who will look after me? Who will pay the money for medical treatment?'* I could not answer her questions and worries. *'I do not want to live many years. I want to die happily, without burdening any one'*, she said.

Case Study 6

Mrs N is 70 years and she has two daughters and two sons. Both the sons and daughters got married and are settled. Her sons are working in Tata Steel Company and staying in the city. Her husband was an agricultural labourer. They had a small piece of land and one small shop. When her husband was alive, they were staying in the village. Most unexpectedly, her husband passed away, leaving her alone.

After her husband's death, she was staying alone in the same village. After her husband's death, her elder son requested her to stay with him. One year she stayed with the elder son and six months with the younger son. She said – *'My sons are good, but daughters-in-law are not that good. In the beginning my daughters-in-law were taking care of me, but gradually they started quarrelling with me on small–small things. Then, I told my son that I want to go back to the village. In the beginning, he was not ready to send me back to the village. But somehow I convinced him telling that someone should be there to look after the house and land'.*

She said – *'Nowadays, everyone wants to stay in a small family of husband, wife and children. Nobody wants their old parents to stay with them. Especially if one becomes widow, then nobody is there to take care of her'.* Sons come to see her every month and give her the required money. One of her grandchildren was staying with her since his childhood. But now he has grown up and got married. Her grandson and his family is living very close to her house. *'Jise chhote se bara kiye wo bhi dekh-bhal nahi karta hai, bahu ke karan muje yanha rahana parta hai, kya kare jeene ke liya to rahana parega na (I have taken care of him for many years, but he is also not taking care of me now. See, I have to stay here alone)'.*

Her nephew was taking care of her land but he never gives money or rice from the land to this old lady. She shares all her problems with one of her neighbours. She cannot walk properly so her neighbour visits her every evening. For vegetables and other requirements, villagers help her. She said – *'Now I do not want to live more. It is better to die rather than stay like this'.* She continued – *'Duniya janti hai ki pati rahne se sabhi puchhte hai baad mein koi nahi puchhta hai, (Everyone knows, if husband is alive then everyone will ask about you, otherwise nobody will even think of you)'.*

When I addressed her calling 'Dadi', she was very happy and offered me lunch which she prepared for herself. I can see the loneliness and helplessness of this old lady. *'Being a widow, I do not have any problem as such. But having two sons and daughters-in-law, still I am staying alone, this makes me feel more depressed'.* Sometimes, even neighbours blame her. *'Why are you staying here alone? You should go and stay with your sons. You have every right to demand help and protection from your adult sons'.*

Case Study 7

Mrs K is 83 years and has two sons and four daughters. She got married in her childhood (she does not even know her exact age during the time of marriage). When she was 15 years old, she came to her in-law's house. She and her husband were working as agricultural labourers. They were cultivating vegetables and selling in the market. She also got 25 katta of land from her father. With this land and hard work, they managed to give education to their children and arranged their marriages. For her daughter's marriage, they have to sell 10 *katta* of land to pay dowry. Her elder son was a vegetable vendor but was not earning enough money to run a house. One day he committed suicide. After that, daughter-in-law took all the land and continues to stay in the house.

Mrs K underwent very difficult times, neglected by family members. Anyhow she made a BPL card with the help of other villagers in her own name. With this BPL card, she is getting 21 kg of rice, 13 kg of wheat, and 3 litres of kerosene. She said – '*Although I am not getting all these items every month, I get rice every month*'. She keeps 5 kg of rice for herself and sells the remaining 16 kg to earn some money. With this money, she is managing her other expenses.

She is not receiving widow pension or old age pension. Even she never applied. '*I cannot do this paper work all alone*'. She had some money saved in her name (₹ 12,000) which she got from her land. She said – '*I cannot use this money because if I use it, then in any emergency happens whom I will ask?*' She cannot expect anything from her son and daughter-in-law. Further she mentioned – '*My daughter-in-law is always quarrelling with me. My son and daughter-in-law are not taking care of me. My neighbours help me*'. In her own words – '*Isi din ko dekhane ke liye itana kast karke bete to aadmee banaye, pr mujhe kya pata that ki beta aisa ho jayega (I have taken all pains to bring up my son. But for whom I was doing all the hard work all these years, now treats me like this!)*'.

One day her son and daughter-in-law started abusing her and started beating her. When her neighbours came to stop them, her son said to them – '*This is our family matter, no need to interfere in our matters*'. Next day, one of her neighbours advised her to complain to the police and then she lodged a complaint against her son and daughter-in-law. Police came and took her son. Her daughter-in-law started threatening the old widow. She went to police station and requested the officer to leave her son. After sometime, her son started beating her again. '*I cannot go to the police station again. Even my neighbours will not help me*'.

She said with tears in her eyes – '*I will die but I will not leave this place*'. She is even worried that her son will question her for talking to 'outsiders and strangers'. *'This house is like a jail. I have no freedom to talk, move and meet people. At least in jail, prisoners get enough food to eat'.*

Case Study 8

Mrs X. is a 65-year-old widow belonging to a tribal family. Five years ago her husband expired due to T.B. She has one son and three daughters. All her children are married. She earns little money by working as a maid in a nearby home. Her husband was unemployed. He used to take all her money for drinking alcohol.

After husband's death, her neighbours started calling her a '*witch*' (*daayan*). Her neighbours do not like her and will not talk to her. She is now considered as 'inauspicious'. Villagers believe that seeing her is a bad omen. They are scared that she can do 'black magic' and hurt people. They want to get rid of her and send her away from the village. *'If you want to be alive, then do not show your face to anyone and stay at home'*. No one is ready to listen to her, because for them she is a 'witch'.

Everyone started blaming her for her husband's death. Because of people's attitude, she could not work outside. She is completely helpless and frustrated. *She asked – 'Do I look like a daayan?'* In her own words – *'Agar kisika pati kam umar main mar gaya to kya wo aurat daayan hoti hai? (If the husband dies at a very young age, does that mean the wife is a witch?)'*.

When I was planning to conduct the survey in that village, some women told me – *'you have to be careful here as some of the widows are witches'*. They know black magic and can harm you, I was told. I just asked them – *'If she does something bad to me, then what I can do?'* They replied – *'In our village there is one tantric, who can help to get rid of black magic. However, it is better for you to avoid meeting those women'*.

When I went to her house for interviewing her, she was courteous. While talking to me she opened up her feelings: 'Everyone in this village think that I am a witch.' She started crying. I asked her – 'Why do people think that you are a witch?' She replied – *'I became a widow before my hair became white, so people believe that I am a witch'*.

Mrs X. was treated as a 'witch' by upper caste families in the village. Widows are blamed here even for their husband's death. People do not want to see them. They are not permitted to attend auspicious ceremonies. In all respect, they are socially and economically 'out casted'. It is a pity that even educated persons in the village believe and support this 'inhuman' practice of branding and treating old widows from lower castes as witches.

Case Study 9

Mrs Y is a widow of 82 years. Her husband expired due to cancer. He was a doctor. After marriage they were happily living in the nearby town. Her husband knew about his health condition, so he saved some money for his wife.

After his death, Mrs Y. came back to her in-law's house in the village. Her brother-in-law was not ready to take her into the family and advised her to go to her own brother's house. She then went to her brother's house in the adjacent village. She stayed there for two years. After two years, she wanted to stay with her brother-in-law's family. But her brother-in-law said – *'You are a widow and how can you stay with us?'* In her own words – *'Vidhava hone ke baad koi apne sasural mein kaise rahega? Hum log tumhare bachche ko rakh sakte hai par pura kharch tumko dena hoga. (After widowhood, how can you stay at your in-law's place? We can keep your son with us but all expenses for him to be given by you)'*. She never expected a reply like this. After hearing this, her own brother said – *'You are my sister and you will never be a burden on us. No need to stay with your brother-in-law. You come with us'*. She stayed with her brother till her son became eleven years old, and then she moved to another village. Her brother made a *pucca* house for her and also gave everything required.

I asked her – *'What made you to move away from your brother's house?'* She replied – *'My brother and sister-in-law are very good persons and really take care of me. But villagers were telling that now I should stay alone. It is not good to stay in 'mayika' (parental house) for rest of the life'*. So she decided to live separately.

Her son has started working in the Block Office as a clerk on a temporary basis. Now she has two grandchildren. Her granddaughter is 15 years old but she is mentally challenged. Her brother also comes to see her frequently and also gives money for monthly expenses. She is receiving widow pension since last one year. She utilizes her pension money for buying cloths, medicines, tonic, Horlicks, etc. She said – '*Now I have no problem at all. But I always wonder, why no one from my husband's family ever enquires about me? How can they treat a daughter-in-law like this?*' Now she has no relationship with them. She learned many lessons in life. For her, her brother-in-law's behaviour was a shock. Fortunately for her, her own brother and his family extended all support. While leaving her, she added – '*Now I realize the worth of siblings. Had my brother not been there, I would have committed suicide long back*'.

Case Study 10

Mrs Z. is a Muslim widow of 64 years. At the age of 18, she got married to her maternal uncle's son who was then 26 years old. He had timber business. They have seven children (four sons and three daughters). Their three sons and one daughter got married. Sons were working in a motor garage. Her husband was very affectionate and caring in the beginning and whatever money he earned, he gave it to his wife. However, he used to consume a lot of alcohol and started spending money for drinks.

One day she came to know from others that her husband has a relationship with another woman, staying near to their house. After few months, her husband started staying with that woman. He never came to see Mrs Z. even when she was sick. When her husband stopped giving money, she started working for her survival. She would go to the jungle to collect wood and then sell it in market. Her husband passed away after a few years.

She asked her brother for some help but he refused – '*I have arranged marriage for you, now it is not my responsibility to look after you. If your husband is not giving money, then how can you expect help from others?*' Her brother suggested her to marry another man. But she did not agree.

Now, she is staying alone and is happy. Few months ago one of her granddaughters started staying with her. Being a widow she has suffered a lot. She said – '*Widow hone ke baad to life aur narak ho jata hai, shadi se pahale to maa-baap ya bhai dekhata hai, lekin shadi ke baad agar pati achcha nahi hai to koi nahi hai puchchane wala! (After widowhood life becomes a hell, before marriage mother or father or brother takes care, but after marriage if husband is not good then nobody will even help you)'.*

She does not know anything about her husband's property. He gave everything to his second wife. She was cursing the second wife – '*She had broken my family, so she will never be happy*'. She is worried for her old age situation. Her children are not taking care of their mother. Now she can do her work but after some years – '*When I become aged and bed-ridden, then nobody is there to look after me. What will happen to me then? Only god can save me*'. I can see the tension and anxiety in her eyes. Like many other widows in the village, she is clueless on what will happen in future.

Appendix B

Key Informant Interviews

1. Head of the Village

Mr W is *mukhiya* of Baharagora Panchayat (Sarpanch) for the last 13 years. There are 22 villages under this gram panchayat. Some of the villages are very much in the interior and it is very difficult to reach there because of poor transportation facility.

Regarding the status of elders in the village, the *mukhiya* said – '*During my young age, we used to give a lot of respect to the elders, but the new generation does not pay any attention towards elders*'. Nowadays the young daughters-in-law are not taking care of their mothers-in-law. The situation is more difficult, in case the woman is a widow. In many families, sons and daughters-in-law never want to support their elderly mother, according to Mr W.

In the villages here, mostly poor widows are working as maids in rich households. People want to keep them as they will not have much responsibility of their children, and they are ready to work at low salary. Another reason of keeping elderly widows as maids is they will work full time without asking extra money. Since they are old, they usually do not go away from the village.

He further mentioned that earlier widows in some of these villages are viewed as '*daayan*' (witch), but now the attitudes of people are changing and they are not blaming widows for the death of their husbands. But still '*daayan pratha*' exists in the community and this is more common among the lower castes. Lower caste widows are having more freedom than those from upper castes. Higher castes are more rigid on their cultural practices and have more restrictions for widows. However, widows from the lower castes can remarry. Even then there is not a single case of remarriage in the village or neighbouring villages. In case any young widows remarry, then she will be thrown out from the village and also from the community.

Mukhiya admitted that many deserving elderly widows are not getting pension. According to him, he went many times to the block level offices enquiring about widow/old age pension. *'How can they be so insensitive to poor old women?'* he asks.

According to him, though there is old age homes in the district, many elderly widows are not interested to go and stay there, even if it is free of cost. *'Old people are so attached to their house and village; they do not want to stay anywhere else. They want to die in the same place where they spent all their life'.* Even well settled children want to take elderly mothers to their place, but women are least interested to move out of the village.

2. Ms Q. (Employee in an old age home located in the study district)

This old age home was established in 1964 by Christian Missionaries. In the beginning, this home was working for the leprosy patients and later became an old age home. Ms Q is working here as a care-taker for the last four years. They pick up the old people from the streets and bring them here so that they can spend their remaining life peacefully and gracefully. Regular prayers are conducted every morning and evening.

Inmates do not have to pay anything for accommodation and food in this old age home. There are 120 inmates now of which 36 are males. Most of the old women are weak and four of them are blind. There are rooms for males and females. The arrangements are such that the bed of one physically dependent elderly is adjacent to another physically independent elderly, so that one can take care of another. Some of them were mentally challenged as they cannot tell anything about themselves. Most of the women in this old age home are widows. They left their houses either because the sons were not taking care of them or daughters-in-law do not want to keep them. There are 12 staff members in this home. In general, all inmates are happy and they feel that now they are living with their family members. This old age home is run with money donated by people. Government also supports to some extent.

The housekeeper of the old age home narrated some incidences about how some elderly widows reached there. In some cases, their children forcefully admitted them here. In other instances, old widows not able to tolerate the harassment at home decided to come here. Irrespective of caste and religion, all were given support, care and attention.

3. Care-Taker of a Private Old Age Home

There are 19 inmates in this private old age home, among them nine are females. For admission to this old age home, each need to deposit ₹ 15,000 and also have to pay ₹ 1,500 every month for accommodation and food. When I asked the care-taker, who is also an inmate, that why he decided to come to old age home, his answer was – '*Jab koi nahi hota hai to kahin to jana hoga*'. He said that I do not have a son and my brother's elder son has taken away all my property. One day he threw me and my wife out to this old age home. My wife was mentally disturbed when we came to this old age home. However, she could not adjust with the situation here.'

I asked – 'How did you manage the money to join here?' He said – 'I had some land that I sold and that was enough to make deposit amount to stay in the old age home'. Further he mentioned – '*What I will do with the land? At least here I am getting enough food. This place is better than my house. I do not want to go back*'.

He narrated incidences in which parents were forcefully brought here by children. One day a young man, who is working in a private company, brought his 80-year-old mother and told me – '*Sir, please keep her here. I will pay whatever you want*'. Another man justified his decision of forcing his mother to be at old age home – 'My mother and wife started quarrelling every day. What can I do?'

Although there is routine life in old age home but some time people come here and distribute sweets and clothes which makes the inmates happy. They are allowed to go out, but they have to take permission from the manager and have to return on time. When ever needed, a doctor will come for check-up.

One widow inmate is very fond of flowers. She developed a garden and spends her time on it. According to her – '*This garden is like my children. I feel very happy when I do gardening*'.

Another old widow revealed the situation which made her an inmate of this old age home. One day her daughter-in-law told her: 'I will show you one place where people like you come and make friends'. She took her and said that tonight you stay here and see how is this place. I stayed one night here and next morning my daughter-in-law said – '*Now you try to stay in this place only. It is very difficult to take care of you. Whenever you need help, we will come here and see you*'.

After few months, she went home to see her grandson, then daughter-in-law said – '*If you come every Sunday, then he will not study. So you need not come every Sunday to spoil my son's future*'. The old lady had no answers.

Each inmate of this old age home has their reasons to be here. They are happy to live with other inmates who share similar feelings. According to the caretaker – '*Many elderly, particularly old widows, are not feeling safe at home. Here, there is a watchman and supporting staff*'. As one inmate said – '*Earlier when I was at home I was feeling very lonely. Now I have many friends here. We not only share our happiness, but also our problems*'.

4. A Doctor in a Government Hospital in the Study Area

According to the medical officer I interviewed, most elderly patients complain about general problems that arise during old age such as joint pain, weakness, etc. Some elderly are suffering from asthma, hypertension and diabetes. Family members do not understand the health requirements of elderly members which demand regular check-up. Sometimes family members bring elderly at the last moment when the health condition is very serious. For those elderly or widows who are staying alone, nobody is worried. Even their children staying in the same village never bothered to find out their health problems.

Old age, widowhood and staying alone add mental tension leading to depression among old widows. Loneliness and depression are common among the elderly widows in the locality.

According to the doctor, the relatives are not ready to spend money for treatment of the aged. According to the doctor, '*When elderly comes alone, we request them to bring some family member along with them*'. Many elderly widows are anaemic as they are poor and cannot afford nutritious food. '*Even the elderly living with their family never come for the routine check-up. Then think about the situation of poor elderly widows and of those who are living alone*'. Family may not be always considerate in dispensing care to the elderly and this is more so when he/she becomes a liability physically and economically. Sometimes, elderly widows come to the hospital with minor problems: '*When I discuss with them, then they start crying stating that nobody takes care of them*'.

Most problems are due to loneliness and fear. There are no psychiatrists in our block. I often console them and make them understand the reality. Sometimes, he provides counselling to patients. But what hurts them most is the way their family members or children behave with them. They realize that they are the most ignored and unwanted persons in the family. Depression gradually leads to more serious health problems. He mentioned – '*This is the responsibility of family members to take care of the elderly or widows. But many family members never worry about their own elderly parents*'. There is a need for opening counselling centres for the aged and widows. Through proper counselling, many psychological and health problems can be minimized to a great extent.

According to the doctor, '*Elderly widows in our villages are the most neglected people. Nobody really cares for them. Once a young man came to my hospital with his 80-year-old mother who had severe health problems. Out of desperation, he told me: "Doctor, I am spending lot of money on my mother's treatment. I think it is good for her and good for me if she leaves this world as early as possible".*'

5. Block Development Officer in the Study Area

During the field work, many elderly widows stated that they are not receiving any pension. Similarly, interviews with Sarpanch also indicated that they do not know why pension applications were rejected. I interviewed a Block Development Officer (BDO) who processes the pension applications.

Few elderly widows are destitutes and many of them are not having knowledge about the procedure to apply for a pension. 'Gram Sevak' identifies the eligible women for pension and also helps them in paper work. Social pension schemes in India are designed to reach out to the destitute elderly, widows and persons with disabilities who have no regular means of subsistence from their own sources of income or through financial support from family members or other sources. Thus, the key eligibility criteria are age, widowhood and destitution. However, interviews with Sarpanch and Block Development Officer indicate that the most commonly used destitution criterion is the possession of a Below Poverty Line card (BPL card) or ration card. Further, he mentioned – '*BPL status used to identify the pension beneficiaries is likely to lead to significant exclusion and inclusion errors*'.

According to the BDO – '*There are many elderly and widows who have applied for pension but we found that they do not have proper documents. Many of them even do not have age proof certificate. Though most of them are eligible to receive pensions, because of lack of proper documents they are not getting it*'. Sometimes it becomes difficult to locate the widows, because they usually move out of the village after the death of their husbands.

For the distribution of money, the officer informed that earlier pension was distributed in cash but now they have opened bank account for all pensioners and directly money goes to their account. It is compulsory for all pensioners that they should have a bank account at the time of submission of application. Block Officer also revealed :

'*There are some problems from the government side. There is a delay in sending the fund. Because of this, many elderly and widows are not getting pension regularly*'. Further he said – '*Now, the number of the elderly is increasing and the number of pensioners has also increased accordingly Administrative procedures take a lot of time. But people do not understand it. Every day elderly come to the Block Office and enquire about their pension. Without having documents, they blame the government*'. On many occasions though we send the list of all eligible women for pension to the concerned departments, but there they bring down the numbers. We can only give pensions to those whose names have been approved by higher authorities.

Few surveyed elderly widows stated that because they are illiterate, it becomes difficult to get papers from the Block Office. Even after the Mukhiya certifies the required documents for pension (age proof, husband's death certificate, income certificates, etc.), then also it is difficult to get the approval of the department concerned.

According to the BDO – *'Many times I feel sad that I could not help the poor aged women. Most of them deserve pension and governmental support. However, they are not able to produce the necessary documents. What can I do?'* When asked about corruption and leakage of pension money, he replied like this – *'We are far better. We deposit the pension into the applicant's bank account. There is very little scope for any official to collect bribe. Tell me, one place or department where there is no corruption?'*

References

Aggarwal, V. and N.K. Chadha, 1990, Hopelessness, Alienation and Life Satisfaction among Aged, Paper Presented at 18th Session of the Indian Science Congress, Indore, 30 January 1990.

Alam, M. and Mukta Mukherjee, 2003, Ageing, ADL Disabilities and Need for Public Health Initiatives, *Discussion Paper Series No. 78/2003,* Institute of Economic Growth, New Delhi.

Alam, M., 2006, *Ageing in India: Socio-Economic and Health Dimensions,* Academic Foundation, New Delhi.

Altekar, A.A., 1973, *The Position of Women in Hindu Civilization: From Prehistoric Times to the Present Day*, Motilal Banarsidass Publishers, New Delhi.

American Psychological Association, 2004, *Elder Abuse and Neglect: In Search of Solutions.* www.apa.org/ageing/elderabuse.html.

Arling, Greg T., 1976, The Elderly Widows and her Family Neighbours and Friends, *Journal of Marriage and the Family*, Vol. 38 (4): 757–768.

Aruna, C. and Chandramohan Reddy, 2001, What Support by Kin to Widows? *Indian Journal of Social Work,* Vol. 62(1): 1–12.

Audinarayana, N. and N. Kavitha, 1997, Living Arrangements of the Widowed and Currently Married Women in Tamil Nadu State, India, in Arvind K. Joshi (ed.), *Older Persons in India*, Serial Publications, New Delhi.

Audinarayana, N., J. Sheela and N. Kavitha, 1997, Are the Elderly Women the Most Deprived among the Deprived? A Micro Level Investigation in Rural Tamil Nadu, in L. Thara Bhai (ed.) *Aging Indian Perspective*, Decent Books, New Delhi.

Balachandran, M., A.S. Raakhee and Sam Sananda Raj H., 2007, Life Satisfaction and Alienation among Elderly Male and Female, *Journal of the Indian Academy of Applied Psychology,* Vol. 33(2): 157–160.

Balkwell, Carolyn, 1981, Transition to Widowhood: A Review of the Literature, *Economic and Political Weekly,* Vol. 30 (1): 117–127.

Bansod, D., 2007, Health, Family and Social Adjustment of Elderly in Rural Maharashtra, Unpublished Ph.D Thesis, International Institute for Population Sciences, Mumbai.

Baron, Omar and Rolf Ehrenfels, 1941, *Mother Rights in India*, Oxford University Press, Hyderabad.

Bell, Hugh M., 1934, *The Adjustment Inventory*, Stanford University Press, California.

Bhagat, B. Ram and Sayeed Unisa, 2006, Ageing Dependency in India: A New Measurement, *Asian Population Studies*, Vol. 2(2): 201–214.

Bhat, P.N. Mari, 1992, Changing Demography of Elderly in India, *Current Science*, Vol. 63 (8, 25): 440–448.

Bhat, P.N. Mari, and R. Kanbargi, 1984, Estimating the Incidence of Widow and Widowers Remarriage in India from Census Data, *Population Studies*, Vol. 38(1): 89–103.

Bhatt, N. Vighnesh, 2006, Status of Widows in Karnataka: Historical Account and Analysis of Present Scenario, in P.K.B. Nayar (ed.) *Widowhood in Modern India*, The Women Press, New Delhi.

Bian, F., 1998, Intergenerational Relations in Urban China: Proximity Contact and Help to Parents, *Demography*, Vol. 35: 115–24.

Bose, A.B. and K.D. Gangrade, 1988, State of Widowhood and Trends in India, in Godavari D. Patil (ed.) *Hindu Widows: A Study in Deprivation,* Gyan Publishing House, New Delhi.

Boss, A.B., 1966, Some Characteristics of Widows in Rural Society, *Man in India*, Vol. 46: 230.

Bruch, Thomas K. and Mathews Beverly J., 1987, Household Formation in Developed Countries, *Population Developments Review*, Vol. 13: 495–511.

Carson, R., J. Butcher and S. Mosby, 2003, *Abnormal Psychology and Modern Life*, Pearson Education Pvt. Ltd., Bangalore.

Census of India, 2001, *Population Census Abstract: Jharkhand*, Series 21 Directorate of Census Operations, Jharkhand.

Census of India, 2001, *Social and Cultural Tables India*, Registrar General and Census Commissioner of India.

Chaudhuri, Anoshua and Kakoli Roy, 2009, Gender Differences in Living Arrangements amongst Older Persons in India, *Journal of Asian and African Studies*, Vol. 44 (3): 259–277.

Chen, F. and S.E. Short, 2008, Household Context and Subjective Well-being among the Oldest-old in China, *Journal of Family Issues*, Vol. 29 (10): 1379–1403.

Chen, M. and J. Dreze, 1992, Widows and Health in Rural India, *Economic and Political Weekly*, Vol. 28 (43 and 44): WS 81–92.

Chen, Martha Alter (ed.), 1998, *Widows in India: Social Neglect and Public Action,* Sage Publications, New Delhi.

Chen, X., and M. Silverstein, 2000, International Social Support and the Psychological Well-being of Older Parents in China, *Research on Aging*, Vol. 22(1): 43–65.

Dandekar, K., 1986, *The Elderly in India*, Sage Publications, New Delhi.

David, R. Phillips, Oi Ling Siu, Anthony G.O. Yeh. and Kevin H.C. Cheng, 2008, Informal Social Support and Older Person's Psychological Well-being in Hong Kong, *Journal of Cross Cultural Gerontology,* Vol. 23: 39–55.

Davis, K. and J. Blake, 1956, Social Structure and Fertility: An Analytic Frame Work, *Economic Development and Cultural Change*, Vol. 4(3): 211–215.

Dong, Xin Qi, Melissa A. Simon, Richard Odwazny and Martin Gorbein, 2008, Depression and Elder Abuse and Neglect among a Community: Dwelling Chinese Elderly Population, *Journal of Elder Abuse & Neglect*, Vol. 20(1): 25–41.

Dreze, Jean, and Amartya Sen, 2002, *India: Development and Participation*, Oxford University Press, New Delhi.

Dreze, Jean, and P.V. Srinivasan, 1997, Widowhood and Poverty in Rural India: Some Inferences from Household Survey Data, *Journal of Development Economics*, Vol. 54: 217–234.

Duval, Elelyn, 1971, *Family Development*, J.B. Lippincott Co., New York.

Ellickson J., 1988, Never the Twain Shall Meet: Ageing Men and Women in Bangladesh, *Journal of Cross-Cultural Gerontology*, Vol. 3:53–56.

Fenech, F. Frederick, 2003, Ethical Issues in Ageing, *Clinical Medicine*, Vol. 3(3): 232–234.

Folta, Jeannette R. and Edith S. Deck, 1987, Black Widows in Rural Zimbabwe, *Journal of Cross-Cultural Gerontology*, Vol. 2(4): 321–342.

Gallagher, D.E., J.N. Breckenridge, L.W. Thompson and J.A. Peterson, 1983, Effects of Bereavement on Indicators of Mental Health in Elderly Widows and Widowers, *Journal of Gerontology*, Vol. 38(5): 565–571.

Government of India, 1999, *National Policy on Older Persons*, Ministry of Social Justice and Empowerment, New Delhi.

Green, E.J., 1977, *Marriage and Family: A Basic Self Instruction*, McGraw Hill Book Co., New York.

Gulati, Leela, 1998, Widowhood and Ageing in India, in Martha Alter Chen (ed.), *Widows in India: Social Neglect and Public Action,* Sage Publications, New Delhi.

Gupta, Indrani, Purnamita Dasgupta and Maneeta Sawhney, 2001, Health of the Elderly in India Some Aspects of Vulnerability, *Discussion Paper Series No. 26/2001,* Institute of Economic Growth, New Delhi.

Halakatti, Meera, 1988, Widowhood: Perspectives and Issues, in H.V. Nagesh, P.S. Nair, and A.P. Katti (eds.), *Widowhood in India,* Janata Shikshana Samiti, Dharwad.

Holmes, J.H. and R.H. Rahe, 1967, The Social Re-adjustments Scale, *Journal of Psychosomatic Research*, Vol. 11: 213–228.

Indira, M.A., 1955, *The Status of Women in Ancient India,* Motilal Banarsidass Publishers, Delhi.

Jamuna, D., 2008, Elderly Women in India: Roles and Status, in Joseph Troisi and Ann Lencyk Pawliczko (eds.), *The Elderly Women in Asia: Her Roles and Positions,* International Institute on Ageing, United Nations, Malta.

Jamuna, D., P.V. Ramamurthy and N.N. Sudha Rani, 1996, Psychosocial Aspects of Elderly Widows, in Vinod Kumar (ed.), *Ageing: Indian Perspective and Global Scenario*, Proceedings of the International Symposium on Gerontology and Seventh Conference of the Association of Gerontology (India), New Delhi: 303–306.

Karve, I., 1968, *Kinship Organization in India*, Asia Publication House, London.

Kelphart, W.M., 1981, *The Family Society and Individual*, Houghton Mifflin Co., Boston.

Kim, Eun-jin, and Loren Geistfeld, 2008, What Makes Older Adults Vulnerable to Exploitation or Abuse? *The Forum for Family and Consumer Issues*, Vol. 13(1): on-line: http://ncsu.edu/ffci/publications/2008/v13nl–2008-spring, accessed on 18.03.2012.

Kitchlu, T.N., 1993, *Widows in India*, Ashish Publishing House, New Delhi.

Kodoth, Praveena and S.I. Rajan 2008, Property and Assets as Economic Security, in S. Irudaya Rajan, Carla Risseeuw and Myrtle Perera (eds.), *Institutional Provisions and Care for the Aged: Perspective from Asia and Europe,* Anthem Press, New Delhi.

Kumari, S. and T.V. Sekher, 2012, Status of Elderly Widows in India, *BOLD*, Vol. 22(2): 6–13.

Kumari, S., and T.V. Sekher, 2010, Elderly in Punjab: Economic Dependency, Health Conditions and Living Arrangements, *Man & Development*, Vol. XXXII (1): 77–88.

Kumari, S.R., 2004, Family Dynamics of Widows, *Indian Journal of Applied Psychology,* Vol. 41: 9–12.

Lalitha, K. and D. Jamuna, 2004, Life Experiences of Elderly Widowers, *Indian Journal of Gerontology*, Vol. 17: 117–126.

Lieberman, M.A. and V.L. Sherman, 1989, The Impact of Self-help Groups on the Mental Health of Widows and Widowers, *American Journal of Orthopsychiatry*, Vol. 56(3): 435–449.

Lopata, H.Z., 1996, *Current Widowhood: Myths and Realities,* Sage, Thousand Oaks, CA.

Martin, L.G. and S.H. Preston, 1994, *Demography of Ageing*, National Academy Press, Washington DC.

Martin, L.G., 1989, Living Arrangements of the Elderly in Fiji, Korea, Malaysia and Philippines, *Demography*, Vol. 26(4): 627–643.

Mehta, Manju, Usha Kulshreshta and Rashmi Chowdhry, 2006, *Indian Widows: Coping Styles, Mental Health and Personal Adjustment,* Pointer Publishers, Jaipur.

Mini, G.K., 2009, Socio-Economic and Demographic Diversity in the Health Status of Elderly People in a Transitional Society, Kerala, India, *Journal of Biosocial Science,* Vol. 41(4): 457–467.

Misra, Seema and Enakshi Ganguly Thukral, 1998, Widows and Property Rights: A Study of Two Villages in Bihar, in Martha Alter Chen (ed.), *Widows in India: Social Neglect and Public Action,* Sage Publications, New Delhi.

Momtaz, Yadollah Abolfathi, Tengku Aizan Hamid, Nurizan Yahaya and Rahimah Ibrahim, 2009, Widowhood and Psychological Well-being among Older Malaysians Mediating Effect of Social Network, *Indian Journal of Social Work*, Vol. 70 (3): 375–390.

Nair, P.T., 1978, *Marriage and Dowry in India,* Minerva Associates, Calcutta.

Nandlal, D.S., R.S. Khatri and R.S. Kadian, 1987, Ageing Problems in the Structural Context, in M.L. Sharma and T.M. Dak (eds.), *Ageing in India,* Ajanta Publications, New Delhi.

Nasreen, Asiya, 2007, Coping with Economic Problems in Old Age and Civil Society's Response, *Indian Journal of Gerontology,* Vol. 21 (3): 324–335.

National Sample Survey Organization, 1998, *The Aged in India: Socio-economic Profile,* (52nd Round), New Delhi.

National Sample Survey Organization, 2006, *Morbidity, Health Care and Condition of the Aged* (60th Round), New Delhi.

O'Bryant, L. Shirley, 1988, Sibling Support and Older Widow's Well-being, *Journal of Marriage and Family*, Vol. 50 (1): 173–183.

Orans, M., 1965, The Santal: A Tribe in Search of a Great Tradition http://www:en.wikipedia.org/wiki/Sarna, accessed on 08.03.2011

Panda, P.K., 1994, *Living Arrangement of the Elderly in Rural Orissa,* Working Paper No. 277, Centre of Development Studies, Thiruvananthapuram.

Panda, P.K., 1997, Living Arrangements of the Elderly in Rural Orissa, *Working Paper,* Centre for Development Studies, Thiruvananthapuram.

Pandya, Rameshwari and Priti Shah, 2006, Problems of Elderly Widows of Baroda-Gujarat, in Arvind K. Joshi (ed.), *Older Persons in India,* Serials Publication, New Delhi.

Patil, Godavari D., 2000, *Hindu Widows: A Study in Deprivation,* Gyan Publishing House, New Delhi.

Prakash, I.J., 1996, Ageing Women: A Liability or an Asset, *Research and Development Journal,* Vol. 2(2): 28–32.

Prakash, I.J., 1998, Maintenance and Competence in Daily Living and Well-being of Elderly, *Research and Development Journal,* Vol. 4(2 and 3): 26–32.

Prakash, I.J., 1999, Living Arrangements of the Elderly in India: Implications for Care Giving, *Ageing and Society,* Vol. 9(3–4): 1–11.

Prakash, I.J., 2000, Adult Women and the Ageing Process, *Ageing and Society,* Vol. 10(3, 4): 31–40.

Prasad, K.V., 1998, The Pension Scheme for Widows in Tamil Nadu, In Martha Chen Alter (ed.), *Widows in India: Social Neglect and Public Action,* Sage Publications, New Delhi.

Prasad, S., 2007, *Life of Elderly in India,* Centre for Development Studies, Thiruvanathapuram, *http://mpra.ub.uni-muenchen.de.*

Pravathy, K.A., 2004, Widowhood: A Gender Perspective, in P. Adinarayana Reddy (ed.) *Problems of Widows in India,* Sarup & Sons, New Delhi.

Priya, Lakshmi, 2007, Condition of Disabled Elderly in India, www.esocialsciences.com, accessed on 30th March 2011

Radha Devi, D., 1987, Work Participation of Widows in India, in H.V. Nagesh, P.S. Nair, and A.P. Katti (eds.), *Widowhood in India,* Janata Shikshana Samiti, Dharwad.

Rajan, S. Irudaya and E.T. Mathew, 2008, *Social Security for the Elderly: Experiences from South Asia,* Routledge, Taylor & Francis Group, NY.

Rajan, S. Irudaya and Sanjay Kumar, 2003, Living Arrangements among Indian Elderly: New Evidence from National Family Health Survey, *Economic and Political Weekly,* Vol. 38 (1): 75–80.

Rajan, S. Irudaya and Sanjay Kumar, 2003, Living Arrangements among Indian Elderly: Evidences from National Family Health Survey, *Economic and Political Weekly,* Vol. 38(1): 75–80.

Rajan, S. Irudaya and Sreerupa, 2008, Disease, Disability and Healthcare Utilization among the Aged, in S. Irudaya Rajan, Carla Risseeuw and Myrtle Perera (eds.), *Institutional Provisions and Care for the Aged: Perspective from Asia and Europe,* Anthem Press, New Delhi.

Rajan, S. Irudaya and Syam Prasad, 2008, Pension and Social Security in India, in S. Irudaya Rajan, Carla Risseeuw and Myrtle Perera (eds), *Institutional Provisions and Care for the Aged: Perspective from Asia and Europe,* Anthem Press, New Delhi.

Rajan, S. Irudaya, C.I. Risseeuw and M. Pereira, 2005, *Care of the Aged: Gender, Institutional Provisions and Social Security in India,* Sage Publications, New Delhi.

Rajan, S. Irudaya, U.S. Mishra, and P.S. Sharma, 1999, *India's Elderly: Burden or Challenge?* Sage Publications, New Delhi.

Ramamurthy, P.V., 1968, An Adjustment Inventory for the Aged, *Indian Journal of Psychology,* Vol. 43: 27–29.

Reddy, P. Adinarayana, 2004, *Problems of Widows in India,* Sarup & Sons Publications, New Delhi.

Reddy, P.H., 1988, Demographic Aspects of Widows in India, in P. Adinarayana Reddy (ed.) *Problems of Widows in India,* Sarup & Sons Publications, New Delhi.

Saraswati, Baidyanath, 1988, The Kashivasi Widows, *Man in India,* Vol. 65(2): 107–120.

Sarkar, Lotika and Narayan Banerjee, 1998, Widows in a Tribal Setting in West Bengal, in Martha Alter Chen (ed.), *Widows in India: Social Neglect and Public Action,* Sage Publications, New Delhi.

Sebastian, D. and T.V. Sekher, 2011, Extent and Nature of Elder Abuse in Indian Families: A Study in Kerala, *Research & Development Journal,* Vol. 17(3): 20–28.

Sekher, T.V., 2005, Socio-economic Dimensions of Old Age Security in India: With Special Reference to Karnataka, *Journal of Social and Economic Development,* Vol. 7(1): 12–28.

Shankardass, Mala Kapur, 2003, Concern for Ageing Women in India, *BOLD,* Vol. 13(3): 19–24.

Shapiro, Adam and Keyes M. Lee Corey, 2008, Marital Status and Social Well-Being: Are the Married Always Better Off? *Social Indicators Research,* Vol. 88: 329–346.

Sheoran, Sushma, S. Vermani, and S. Darshan, 2004, Health Problems of Aged Widows in Rural Haryana, *Ageing and Society,* 14 (1 and 2): 47–67.

Sheykhi, Mohammad Taghi, 2006, A Sociological Review of the Reflections and Dimensions of Quality of Life of the Widows in Tehran, *Social Indicators Research,* Vol. 78(2): 251–270.

Sijuwade, O. Philip, 2008, Adjustment of the Elderly in Relation to Living Arrangement, Gender and Family Life Satisfaction, *Pakistan Journal of Social Sciences,* Vol. 5(6): 602–605.

Sijuwade, O. Philip, 2008, Coping with Economic Problems in Old Age and Civil. Society's Response, *Pakistan Journal of Social Sciences,* Vol. 5(7): 691–695.

Singh, Gurmeet, 1986, Problems of Widowhood, *The Indian Journal of Social Work*, Vol. XLVII, (1): 67–75.

Siva Raju, S., 2011, *Studies on Ageing in India: A Review*, Working Paper Series on Ageing, Institute for Social and Economic Change (ISEC), Bangalore.

Sivagami, A. and M. Thamilrasan, 2004, Empowering Widows for Development, in P. Adinarayana Reddy (ed.) *Problems of Widows in India,* Sarup & Sons Publications, New Delhi.

Soodan, K.S., 1975, *Ageing in India*, Department of Social Work, University of Lucknow, Lucknow.

Srinivas, P., 1982, Problems of the Aged in India, *Yojana*, Vol. 46(10): 1–15.

Stark, John R., 1954, Economic Status of Older People, *The Journal of Business*, Vol. 27(2): 119–130.

Sureender, S., M. Vaithilingam and A.G. Khan, 1996, Distress of the Aged Widows in Rural Tamil Nadu, *Research and Development Journal*, Vol. 2(2): 41–46.

Thara Bhai, L. 2004, *Widows in India*, B.R. Publishing Corporation, New Delhi.

Troisi, J., 2000, *Tribal Religion*, Manohar Publishers, New Delhi.

Truxual, Andrew G. and E. Merrill Francis, 1953, *Marriage and the Family in American Culture*, Prentice-Hall Inc, Englewood Cliffs, NJ.

UNFPA, 1998, *The State of World Population–1998*, United Nations Population Fund, New York.

United Nations, 2001, *Widowhood: Invisible Women, Secluded or Excluded, Woman 2000 and Beyond*, Division for the Advancement of Women, United Nations.

United Nations, 2002, *Gender Dimensions of Ageing: Women 2000*, Department of Economic and Social Affairs, United Nations, New York.

United Nations, 2002, *World Population Ageing 1950–2050*, Population Division, Department of Economic and Social Affairs, New York.

United Nations, 2006, *World Population Prospects*, Population Division, Department of Economic and Social Affairs, New York.

Velkof, Victoria A., 2001, Living Arrangements and Well-Being of the Older Population: Future Research Direction, *Population Bulletin of the United Nations,* Special Issues No. 42/43 (3–4): 376–385.

Vyas, S. and Lilani Kumaranayake, 2006, *Constructing Socio-Economic Status Indices: How to Use Principal Components Analysis*, London School of Hygiene and Tropical Medicine, London, UK.

Waweru, L.M., E.W. Kabiru, J.N. Mbithi and E.S. Some, 2003, Health Status and Health Seeking Behaviour of the Elderly Persons in Dagoretti Division, Nairobi, *East African Medical Journal*, Vol. 80 (2): 63–68.

Wu, Z. and C.M. Schimmele, 2008, Living Arrangements and Psychological Disposition of the Oldest Old Population in China, in Y. Zeng, D.L. Poston, Jr. D.A. Vlosky and D.Gu Dordrecht (eds.), *Healthy Longevity in China: Demographic, Socio-economic, and Psychological Dimensions*, Springer, Netherlands.

Yadava, K.N.S., 2011, Attitude and Behaviour of Family Members and Satisfaction of Elderly: Some Related Issues, in K.N.S. Yadava and Alok Kumar (eds.), *Ageing-Some Emerging Issues: Profiles, Trends and Policy Perspectives*, Manak Publications Ltd., New Delhi.

Yesavage, J.A. Brink, T.L Rose, T.L. Lum O, V. Huang, M.B. Adey and V.O. Leirer, 1983, Development and Validation of a Geriatric Depression Screening Scale: A Preliminary Report, *Journal of Psychiatric Research*, Vol. 17: 37–49.

Zimmer, Zachary and Julia Kwong, 2003, Family Size and Support of Older Adults in Urban and Rural China: Current Effects and Future Implications. *Demography*, Vol. 40(1): 23–44.

Index